Insulin Stability

Blood Sugar, Insulin Resistance, and Metabolic Health

Nathan Reed

PERENNIAL PUBLISHING

Published by Perennial Publishing

Paperback ISBN: 978-1-971996-36-3
Hardcover ISBN: 978-1-971996-37-0
E-book ISBN: 978-1-971996-38-7

Contents

Interpreting Metabolic Systems

Metabolic systems are often interpreted through isolated events. A rise in signaling, a meal, a period without input, or a single observable response is treated as though it defines the behavior of the system. This framing assigns explanatory weight to individual moments while separating them from the conditions that surround them. The limitation is not that events are irrelevant, but that they do not carry sufficient meaning on their own. A signal does not determine outcomes without reference to the state into which it enters. When events are treated as self-contained, the continuity required to understand system behavior is removed, leaving fragments that appear decisive but are structurally incomplete.

A metabolic signal is always part of an ongoing sequence. It arises from an existing baseline, contributes to cumulative exposure, interacts with prior signals, and alters the conditions under which subsequent signals are interpreted. The meaning of any moment is therefore inseparable from its position within this sequence. A rise in signaling may appear significant when viewed in isolation, but its effect depends on whether it follows a period of low exposure or occurs within a persistently elevated baseline. A period without input may appear distinct, yet its interpretive value depends on the timing and structure of prior signals. Without continuity across time, signals lose context, and without context, interpretation becomes distorted.

This limitation of event-based thinking becomes more pronounced in systems governed by signaling relationships. Insulin does not operate as an isolated force acting upon passive tissues. It functions as part of a signaling network in which information is continuously generated, transmitted, and interpreted. The presence of a signal does not define its effect. The effect emerges from how that signal is interpreted within the system. Interpretation depends on conditions such as baseline level, cumulative exposure, responsiveness across tissues, and the structure of timing that organizes signals into patterns. A signal without interpretation is incomplete, and interpretation without context is unstable.

Understanding insulin as information rather than as a direct cause shifts the framework through which metabolic behavior is viewed. A signal conveys a condition—in this case, the availability of energy within the system—but it does not impose a fixed outcome. Different tissues interpret the same signal according to their roles and current state. Muscle may translate the signal into uptake and utilization, liver into regulation of circulating availability, and adipose tissue into allocation and buffering. These responses are not inherent properties of the signal alone. They are outcomes of interpretation, shaped by sensitivity, prior exposure, and the alignment of signaling conditions across tissues.

Because interpretation depends on context, identical signals can produce different responses under different conditions. A signal emerging within a low baseline environment with clear temporal separation may be interpreted distinctly from the same signal occurring within a high baseline environment where signals overlap. The difference is not in the signal itself but in the structure within which it is embedded. This distinction separates signal presence from system behavior and removes the assumption that magnitude alone determines outcome. Magnitude contributes to the pattern, but it does not define it.

The system operates through patterns rather than through isolated events. Patterns are formed by the interaction of magnitude, duration, frequency, sequence, and overlap across time. A signal of moderate magnitude sustained over a longer duration contributes differently to system behavior than a brief signal of higher magnitude. Frequent signals with incomplete resolution produce a different interpretive environment than less frequent signals that allow full separation. Sequence determines whether signals reinforce or counterbalance one another, and overlap determines whether distinct states remain distinguishable or merge into continuous exposure. These elements do not operate independently. They combine to form patterns that the system interprets as a whole.

Exposure emerges from the interaction of these patterns across time. It reflects the cumulative presence of signaling across time, shaped by how often signals occur, how long they persist, and how completely they resolve. Baseline emerges as a related property, representing the reference level from which new signals are interpreted. Variability defines the structure of fluctuation around that baseline, determining whether oscillation remains organized or becomes irregular. Together, baseline, exposure, and variability define system state. They establish the conditions within which signals are interpreted and responses are generated.

System state is not static. It is continuously shaped by prior signaling patterns. This introduces path-dependence, where current interpretation reflects accumulated conditions rather than only present inputs. A system operating with low baseline and structured variability interprets signals differently than a system operating with elevated baseline and disorganized fluctuation. The same input modifies these systems in different ways because it enters different interpretive environments. Inputs do not act independently of state. They interact with it, modifying patterns that are already in motion.

This interaction between inputs and state reinforces the need to move beyond event-based reasoning. A single input does not determine outcome because it cannot override the structure into which it enters. Nutrition, fasting, and stress influence the system by altering timing, exposure, baseline, and variability, but their effects depend on how these variables are already configured. A period of reduced signaling may contribute to clearer separation under one set of conditions and have minimal effect under another. A change in input timing may reorganize pattern structure in one context and introduce variability in another. The significance of any input is therefore conditional, shaped by the system rather than imposed upon it.

Within this framework, insulin must be positioned without evaluative bias. It is not inherently beneficial or harmful, and it does not function as a target to be maximized or minimized. It is a coordination signal that communicates energy availability and participates in aligning tissue-level responses within the broader system. Its role is informational. It reflects conditions and contributes to their organization. When interpretation is clear and coordination is preserved, signaling supports stable behavior. When the signaling environment is altered, the same signal participates in distorted patterns. The difference lies not in the signal itself but in the structure of the system within which it operates.

Removing moral framing from insulin is necessary to preserve analytical clarity. Assigning value to the signal obscures the conditions that determine its interpretation. It shifts attention away from pattern formation, state, and interaction across variables, and places it on the signal as an isolated object. This reduction limits the ability to understand how stability and instability emerge. Stability is not a property of insulin alone. It is a property of alignment across timing, sensitivity, clearance, exposure, baseline, variability, and coordination. Instability is not caused by the presence of a signal but emerges when these variables become misaligned, altering how signals are interpreted and how responses are coordinated.

The purpose of this book is to define that system of relationships. It operates as a model of how metabolic behavior emerges from interacting variables rather than as a set of instructions for modifying behavior. It does not provide protocols, prescribe actions, or frame outcomes as goals. It explains how signaling functions, how interpretation shapes response, and how patterns across time determine system behavior. Mechanisms are presented to clarify relationships, not to direct application. The distinction is structural rather than practical. Explanation precedes any consideration of use, and interpretation precedes any attempt at modification.

Approaching the system requires a shift in how information is read. Individual mechanisms are not intended to stand alone as explanations of behavior. They are components of a network that only becomes coherent when their interactions are considered together. Timing cannot be understood without reference to clearance and exposure. Sensitivity cannot be interpreted without considering baseline and variability. Coordination cannot be separated from how signals are interpreted across tissues within a shared environment. Reading for isolated conclusions fragments the system, while reading for relationships allows its structure to emerge.

This relational approach changes the level at which understanding occurs. Instead of focusing on discrete outcomes, attention shifts to how variables interact across time to produce those outcomes. Instead of identifying singular causes, the system is understood as a set of conditional relationships. Instead of treating inputs as determinants, they are seen as modifiers of pattern structure. The emphasis moves from what happens in a moment to how moments are connected, from what a signal is to how it is interpreted, and from what appears to occur to how it is generated through interaction.

Within this perspective, metabolic stability is not defined by the absence of change. It is defined by the presence of structured change that remains interpretable and coordinated across variables. Signals vary, patterns evolve, and conditions shift, but alignment across timing, sensitivity, baseline, exposure, variability, and coordination preserves the system's ability to maintain coherent behavior. When that alignment is reduced, interpretation becomes less precise, responses become less coordinated, and variability becomes less structured. Stability and instability are therefore not separate states but expressions of how effectively the system maintains alignment within its operating conditions.

This introduction establishes the interpretive lens through which the system is understood. It replaces isolated events with continuous patterns, replaces direct causation with interpretation, and replaces single-variable explanations with interaction across variables. It positions insulin as a neutral coordination signal embedded within a network of relationships, and it defines metabolic behavior as the product of those relationships unfolding across time. The system becomes visible not through individual signals but through the structure of their interaction, and understanding emerges from recognizing how patterns, state, and interpretation combine to shape outcomes within a continuously adjusting system.

The Signal Interpretation Mechanism

The Signal Interpretation Mechanism begins with a reframing that removes insulin from the category of substances that act directly on the body and places it within the domain of information that the body interprets. This shift is not semantic. It changes the structure through which metabolic behavior is understood. When insulin is treated as a substance, it is assumed to exert force in a linear and deterministic way, producing outcomes through direct action. When insulin is treated as a signal, it becomes part of a communication system in which meaning is not contained solely within the signal itself, but emerges through interpretation within a dynamic and context-dependent network.

Insulin does not move glucose by force. It does not impose storage as an independent directive detached from surrounding conditions. It communicates the presence, pattern, and temporal characteristics of energy availability. The metabolic system receives this communication and integrates it with concurrent signals, prior states, and current constraints. What follows is not a fixed outcome, but a coordinated response shaped by interpretation. The Signal Interpretation Mechanism defines this process as the central layer through which insulin participates in metabolic regulation. Interpretation, in this context, is the process by which a given insulin signal is translated into a conditional response based on current system state, concurrent signals, and prior exposure history.

The distinction between signal and substance is foundational. A substance operates through direct interaction, where its presence produces a consistent and predictable effect regardless of context. A signal operates through meaning, where its effect depends on how it is interpreted within a system that is already active, already conditioned, and already responding to multiple inputs. Insulin belongs to the second category. Its presence does not dictate a single outcome. Instead, it modifies the informational environment in which decisions are made at the cellular and systemic level.

This distinction becomes visible when considering that identical concentrations of insulin can produce different metabolic outcomes under different conditions. If insulin were functioning as a substance, its effect would be uniform across contexts. The variability observed in metabolic responses indicates that insulin's role is mediated through interpretation rather than direct causation. The same signal can lead to different allocations of energy, different rates of uptake, and different patterns of storage depending on how it is received and processed by tissues operating under specific states.

The interpretation of insulin occurs within a system that is continuously active. Cells do not wait passively for insulin to arrive before determining their behavior. They maintain ongoing processes related to energy use, maintenance, and repair. Insulin enters this environment as additional information, modifying the probabilities of certain actions rather than enforcing them unconditionally. The response is therefore contingent. It reflects both the signal itself and the internal condition of the system at the moment of reception.

This conditionality is central to the Signal Interpretation Mechanism. Tissues do not respond to insulin in isolation. They respond to insulin as part of a broader signaling landscape that includes counter-regulatory hormones, substrate availability, neural input, and circadian modulation. The meaning of insulin is shaped by this landscape. A given signal may indicate abundance under one set of conditions and insufficient coordination under another. Interpretation is therefore not static. It evolves with the system.

The concept of interpretation introduces a temporal dimension that is absent in substance-based models. Signals are not only defined by their magnitude but also by their timing, frequency, and pattern over time. Insulin does not function as a singular event. It operates as part of a sequence of signals that create patterns of exposure. These patterns are interpreted by tissues as indicators of recurring conditions. Over time, the system adapts to these patterns, adjusting its sensitivity, responsiveness, and allocation strategies.

This adaptive process demonstrates that interpretation is not limited to immediate response. It extends into the shaping of future behavior. Repeated signaling patterns influence how subsequent signals are understood. A system exposed to frequent insulin signaling may interpret the same signal differently than a system exposed to intermittent signaling. The difference is not in the signal itself but in the history of interpretation that precedes it. This history alters the context in which new signals are received.

The Signal Interpretation Mechanism therefore includes both acute and chronic dimensions. Acutely, insulin provides information about current energy availability. Chronically, it contributes to the formation of interpretive frameworks that shape how future signals are processed. These frameworks are not conscious. They are embedded within cellular and systemic behavior, expressed through changes in receptor sensitivity, signaling pathways, and substrate handling. The system learns through exposure, and this learning influences subsequent interpretation.

Within this framework, tissues act as interpretive units. They do not respond uniformly. Each tissue integrates insulin with its own functional role, energetic demands, and current state. Muscle tissue, adipose tissue, and hepatic tissue all receive the same signal, but they interpret it through different operational contexts. These contexts determine how the signal is translated into action. The result is coordinated behavior across tissues, not because insulin imposes uniformity, but because each tissue aligns its response with both the signal and its role within the system.

Coordination emerges from distributed interpretation rather than centralized control. Insulin does not direct each tissue independently. It provides a shared informational reference point. Tissues use this reference point to adjust their behavior in ways that maintain overall system stability. This distributed model allows for flexibility. It enables the system to adapt to varying conditions without requiring rigid control mechanisms. Interpretation allows for variation within coordination, preserving both responsiveness and stability.

The variability of interpretation also explains why metabolic outcomes cannot be reduced to single variables. When insulin is viewed as a substance, it becomes tempting to attribute outcomes directly to its presence or absence. This approach ignores the interpretive layer and leads to simplified models that fail to account for observed complexity. By contrast, the signal-based model recognizes that outcomes are the result of interactions between signals, states, and histories. Insulin contributes to these interactions, but it does not determine them independently.

Misinterpretation arises when insulin is treated as a substance rather than a signal. This conceptual error leads to the assumption that insulin directly causes storage, directly inhibits release, or directly determines metabolic state. These assumptions bypass the interpretive layer and reduce a dynamic system to a set of linear relationships. The result is a model that cannot accommodate variability, context, or adaptation. It produces conclusions that appear consistent in isolated scenarios but fail under broader conditions.

The consequences of this misinterpretation extend beyond conceptual error. When insulin is treated as a substance, interventions are often framed around altering its presence without considering how the system interprets that presence. This approach assumes that modifying the signal will produce predictable outcomes, ignoring the fact that interpretation may change in response to both the intervention and the underlying system state. The mismatch between expectation and outcome reflects the absence of the interpretive framework.

Failure patterns emerge when the signal-based nature of insulin is not recognized. One pattern involves the assumption of direct causality, where insulin is seen as the sole driver of specific outcomes. This leads to models that attribute complex behaviors to single variables, neglecting the interactions that define system behavior. Another pattern involves the neglect of temporal dynamics, where the timing and pattern of signaling are overlooked in favor of static measurements. This obscures the role of repetition and adaptation in shaping interpretation.

A further failure pattern involves the neglect of system state. Interpretation depends on the condition of the system at the moment of signaling. Factors such as prior exposure, current energy availability, and concurrent signals all influence how insulin is understood. Ignoring these factors leads to inconsistent predictions, as the same signal produces different outcomes under different conditions. The variability is not random. It reflects differences in interpretation that are not accounted for in substance-based models.

The Signal Interpretation Mechanism addresses these failure patterns by restoring the role of context. It defines insulin as a component of a communication system in which meaning is constructed through interaction. This construction is influenced by multiple layers, including immediate conditions, prior exposure, and system-wide coordination. By incorporating these layers, the mechanism provides a framework for understanding variability without reducing it to noise or error.

Within this framework, stability is not achieved through the elimination of variability but through the management of interpretation. The system maintains stability by interpreting signals in ways that preserve functional balance across changing conditions. This requires continuous adjustment. It requires the ability to integrate new information with existing structures. The Signal Interpretation Mechanism defines this process as the basis of metabolic regulation at the signaling level.

The transition from substance-based to signal-based framing alters how metabolic processes are understood at every level. It shifts the focus from isolated variables to interactions. It replaces direct causality with conditional response. It introduces time as a defining factor in system behavior. Most importantly, it recognizes that outcomes emerge from interpretation rather than from the signal alone. Insulin becomes part of a larger conversation within the body, one that is ongoing, context-dependent, and shaped by the history of prior exchanges.

This conversation is not static. It evolves as conditions change. Signals are produced, received, and interpreted continuously. The meaning of each signal is influenced by what has come before and what is occurring simultaneously. The Signal Interpretation Mechanism captures this dynamic, providing a structure through which metabolic behavior can be understood as the result of coordinated communication rather than isolated action.

By defining insulin as information, the mechanism establishes a foundation for examining how signaling patterns influence system behavior over time. It allows for the analysis of how repeated exposures shape interpretation, how context modifies response, and how coordination emerges from distributed processing. It also clarifies why simplified models fail, as they omit the interpretive layer that determines how signals are translated into action.

The Signal Interpretation Mechanism therefore operates as a central organizing principle. It does not replace existing knowledge about insulin's role in metabolism. It reorganizes that knowledge within a framework that accounts for variability, context, and time. It provides a lens through which metabolic stability and instability can be examined as outcomes of signaling dynamics rather than as direct effects of isolated factors.

In this framework, insulin is no longer positioned as a force that acts upon the body. It is understood as a signal that participates in a network of communication. Its role is to inform, not to impose. The system responds to this information through interpretation, integrating it with other signals and conditions to produce coordinated behavior. This process defines how metabolic systems maintain stability under changing conditions, and how deviations from this process lead to instability.

The Signal Interpretation Mechanism establishes that understanding insulin requires understanding how information is processed within the metabolic system. It requires attention to context, to timing, and to history. It requires recognition that outcomes are not dictated by signals alone but emerge from the way those signals are interpreted within a dynamic and adaptive system.

The Coordination Mechanism

The Coordination Mechanism defines how insulin functions not as an isolated actor within a single tissue, but as a system-wide signal that organizes the distribution and use of energy across multiple domains simultaneously. Its role is not confined to initiating uptake or enforcing storage within a specific location. It operates as a coordinating input that aligns the behavior of muscle, liver, and adipose tissue within a shared informational context. This alignment allows the metabolic system to maintain continuity under changing conditions by ensuring that energy is routed in a manner consistent with current availability, prior exposure, and ongoing demand. Coordination, in this context, is the process by which a shared insulin signal produces aligned but tissue-specific energy routing decisions based on system state, tissue role, and prior signaling patterns.

Coordination begins with the recognition that no tissue operates independently. Each participates in a continuous exchange of substrates and signals, contributing to a system that must balance immediate requirements with longer-term stability. Insulin enters this system as a signal that communicates the presence and pattern of energy availability. Its influence is expressed not through direct action, but through the way it alters the interpretive environment across tissues. Each tissue receives the same signal, but the outcome is determined by how that signal is integrated within its functional role and current state.

The Coordination Mechanism therefore depends on distributed interpretation. Muscle tissue, hepatic tissue, and adipose tissue do not wait for explicit instruction beyond the signal itself. They interpret insulin within the context of their responsibilities and constraints. Muscle tissue evaluates insulin relative to its ongoing energy demands and its capacity to take up and utilize circulating substrates. The liver interprets insulin in relation to its role in regulating circulating energy levels, managing both release and storage across time. Adipose tissue interprets insulin as part of its function in buffering energy availability, adjusting its behavior to maintain stability across periods of fluctuation. These interpretations occur simultaneously, producing coordinated outcomes without centralized control.

This distributed coordination allows for flexible routing of energy. Insulin does not direct energy into a single pathway. It modifies the probabilities associated with multiple pathways, allowing the system to allocate resources based on current conditions. Under certain conditions, a greater proportion of circulating energy may be directed toward immediate use within muscle tissue. Under other conditions, routing may favor hepatic processing or storage within adipose tissue. The signal itself remains consistent in its role as an indicator of availability, but the routing outcome varies as a function of interpretation across tissues.

Energy routing provides a more accurate framework than storage when describing insulin's function. Storage is one possible outcome of coordination, but it is not the defining purpose. The system must continuously decide where energy should be directed at any given moment. These decisions are not binary. They involve gradients of allocation that reflect both the magnitude and pattern of signaling. Insulin contributes to this process by indicating that energy is available for distribution. The system then determines how that energy is routed, balancing immediate use, buffering, and deferred allocation.

The distinction between routing and storage becomes evident when considering that storage is conditional. It occurs when the system interprets that current availability exceeds immediate requirements and that buffering is necessary for future stability. This interpretation is not solely dependent on the presence of insulin. It depends on the interaction between insulin and other signals, as well as the state of the tissues involved. When muscle tissue has capacity for uptake and utilization, routing may favor that pathway even in the presence of insulin signaling that would otherwise support storage. When hepatic regulation indicates a need to maintain circulating levels, routing may shift accordingly. Storage emerges when the system determines that routing toward accumulation supports overall stability.

The liver occupies a central position within this coordination, not as a controlling entity, but as a regulatory interface between input and circulation. It interprets insulin in conjunction with other signals to determine whether to release or retain substrates. Its role in maintaining circulating energy levels requires it to adjust continuously, balancing incoming and outgoing flows. Insulin influences this balance by modifying how the liver interprets the current state of availability. The liver's response contributes to the overall coordination by shaping the substrate environment that other tissues encounter.

Muscle tissue contributes through its capacity to absorb and utilize energy. Its interpretation of insulin is influenced by its current activity level, prior exposure, and internal demand. When demand is elevated, muscle tissue may interpret insulin as an opportunity to increase uptake and utilization. When demand is reduced, its response may shift, altering how much energy is directed toward immediate use versus other pathways. This variability illustrates that coordination is not imposed uniformly. It emerges from tissue-specific interpretation aligned within a shared signaling context.

Adipose tissue functions as a buffering system, adjusting its behavior to maintain stability across fluctuations in availability. Its interpretation of insulin reflects its role in managing surplus and supporting continuity during periods of reduced input. When the system interprets that buffering is necessary, adipose tissue participates by adjusting its uptake and release dynamics. This participation is not independent. It is coordinated with the responses of muscle and liver, ensuring that energy distribution remains aligned with system requirements.

The Coordination Mechanism therefore integrates these tissue-specific responses into a coherent system-level outcome. Coherence does not require uniformity. It requires alignment within a shared informational framework. Insulin provides part of this framework by signaling energy availability, but coordination depends on how this signal interacts with other inputs and how it is interpreted across tissues. The resulting behavior reflects a balance between competing demands, adjusted continuously as conditions change.

Temporal dynamics play a critical role in this process. Coordination is not determined by a single signal event. It evolves through patterns of signaling over time. Repeated exposure to certain patterns influences how tissues interpret subsequent signals, altering their responsiveness and shaping routing decisions. These adaptations are not uniform across tissues. Each adjusts according to its role and exposure history, contributing to a system that evolves in its coordination strategy.

This time-based behavior introduces variability that cannot be captured through static models. The same level of insulin signaling may produce different routing outcomes depending on the recent history of signaling patterns. A system that has been exposed to frequent signals may interpret a given signal differently than one that has experienced intermittent exposure. These differences are expressed through changes in how energy is distributed, demonstrating that coordination is influenced by both current signals and prior conditions.

The Coordination Mechanism also reflects the interaction between signaling and constraint. The system operates within limits defined by capacity, demand, and environmental conditions. Insulin contributes to coordination by providing information about availability, but the system's response is shaped by these constraints. When capacity for uptake is limited within a tissue, routing may shift toward alternative pathways. When demand increases, routing may favor immediate use. These adjustments occur through interpretation, aligning behavior with both the signal and the constraints present.

Coordination extends beyond the distribution of energy at a single moment. It includes the maintenance of stability across time. The system must ensure that energy is not only allocated appropriately in the present but also managed in a way that supports future conditions. This requires balancing immediate use with buffering and deferred allocation. Insulin participates in this balancing process by influencing how tissues interpret current availability in relation to anticipated needs. The outcome is a dynamic equilibrium that adjusts as conditions evolve.

Distortion occurs when coordination becomes misaligned. This misalignment can arise from alterations in signaling patterns, changes in tissue responsiveness, or shifts in system constraints. When tissues interpret insulin in ways that are not aligned with overall system requirements, routing decisions become inconsistent. Energy may be directed toward pathways that do not support stability, leading to accumulation in some domains and insufficiency in others. These imbalances reflect a breakdown in coordination rather than a failure of the signal itself.

One form of distortion involves the decoupling of tissue responses. When muscle, liver, and adipose tissue no longer interpret signals in a coordinated manner, their actions diverge. This divergence disrupts the balance of energy distribution, producing variability that the system cannot easily reconcile. Another form involves the persistence of routing patterns that no longer match current conditions. When prior adaptations continue to influence interpretation despite changes in environment or demand, coordination becomes misaligned with reality.

These distortion patterns highlight that coordination depends on the integrity of interpretation across tissues. Insulin provides a shared signal, but coordination requires that this signal be integrated consistently within the system. When interpretation becomes fragmented, the signal loses its ability to align tissue behavior. The resulting instability is not due to the presence of insulin itself but to the breakdown of the interpretive processes that enable coordination.

The Coordination Mechanism therefore defines insulin's role as part of a distributed system that organizes energy routing through shared information. It establishes that outcomes are determined not by the signal in isolation but by how that signal is interpreted across tissues operating under specific conditions. This interpretation produces coordinated behavior that supports stability when aligned and instability when disrupted.

By focusing on routing rather than storage, the mechanism clarifies that the primary function of insulin is to influence how energy moves through the system. Storage becomes one of several possible outcomes, contingent on the interpretation of current conditions. This framing allows for a more accurate understanding of how metabolic behavior emerges from signaling dynamics, emphasizing that coordination is an ongoing process shaped by context, time, and interaction.

The Coordination Mechanism integrates these elements into a model in which insulin operates as a system-wide coordinator. It does not act upon tissues independently. It provides information that tissues use to align their behavior within a shared framework. This alignment produces the routing patterns that define metabolic function, demonstrating that coordination determines system behavior through the continuous interaction of signals, states, and responses.

The Timing Mechanism

The Timing Mechanism defines how the placement of insulin signaling within time determines its meaning within the metabolic system. Insulin does not function as an isolated event whose effect is determined solely by its magnitude. It operates as part of a sequence of signals, where each instance is interpreted in relation to what precedes it, what follows it, and the intervals that separate it from other signals. The system does not respond to insulin as a discrete input detached from temporal context. It responds to insulin as an element within a structured sequence, and this sequence defines the conditions under which coordination occurs.

Timing establishes the conditions of interpretation. A signal arriving at one point within a sequence may produce a different response than an identical signal arriving at another point. This difference does not arise from a change in the signal itself but from a change in the context created by prior signals and the time intervals between them. The Timing Mechanism therefore shifts the focus from magnitude to placement. It defines insulin not as a quantity that produces effects through its level, but as information whose meaning is shaped by when it appears within an ongoing pattern.

The distinction between sequence and magnitude is central to this mechanism. Magnitude describes the amplitude of a signal at a given moment. Sequence describes the arrangement of signals across time, including their order, spacing, and recurrence. While magnitude contributes to interpretation, it does not define it independently. The same magnitude can be interpreted differently depending on its position within a sequence. A signal of a given amplitude may be understood as a continuation of a prior state, a transition between states, or a disruption of an established pattern, depending on when it occurs.

Sequence introduces relational meaning. Each signal is evaluated in the context of preceding signals, creating continuity or contrast that shapes interpretation. When signals occur in close succession, they may be interpreted as part of a sustained state. When separated by longer intervals, they may be interpreted as distinct events. These interpretations influence how tissues coordinate their responses, altering routing decisions and modifying system behavior. The temporal structure of signaling therefore acts as a framework within which magnitude is interpreted rather than as a secondary characteristic.

Signals do not exist in isolation across time. They interact through overlap, succession, and spacing. This interaction creates patterns that the system learns to recognize and respond to. A series of signals with consistent spacing may establish a stable pattern that tissues interpret as a recurring condition. Irregular spacing may disrupt this pattern, requiring continuous recalibration of interpretation. The system is sensitive not only to the presence of signals but to the structure of their arrangement across time.

Prior signals influence the interpretation of subsequent signals through residual effects on system state. After a signal is received and interpreted, the system does not return immediately to a neutral baseline. It carries forward a modified state that reflects the prior interaction. This state affects how new signals are understood. A signal arriving during a period of residual activity may be integrated differently than the same signal arriving after a period of relative quiescence. The Timing Mechanism accounts for this continuity by recognizing that interpretation is cumulative rather than reset-based.

This cumulative process creates temporal layering. Each signal contributes to a layered context in which multiple past signals influence current interpretation. The system integrates these layers to determine how to respond, producing outcomes that reflect the combined effect of recent and more distant signals. The depth of this layering depends on the duration and intensity of prior sequences, as well as the intervals between them. Timing therefore shapes not only immediate response but the structure of interpretive memory within the system.

Identical signals can carry different meanings depending on timing because they enter the system under different layered conditions. A signal following a sequence of similar signals may reinforce an existing pattern, leading to continuity in response. The same signal following a period of reduced signaling may initiate a transition, prompting a different set of responses. The difference is not in the signal itself but in the temporal context in which it is interpreted. Timing alters meaning by modifying the conditions under which interpretation occurs.

This temporal dependence extends across tissues, influencing coordination. Muscle, liver, and adipose tissue interpret signals within their own temporal contexts, shaped by their recent exposure and internal state. When timing patterns are consistent across tissues, coordination emerges through aligned interpretation. When timing patterns differ, coordination becomes more complex, as tissues may respond to the same signal with differing priorities. The Timing Mechanism integrates these tissue-level dynamics into system-wide behavior by linking temporal patterns to distributed interpretation.

Coordination over time requires that signals form sequences that can be integrated across tissues. These sequences establish expectations within the system, allowing tissues to anticipate and align their responses. When signals follow consistent temporal patterns, tissues adjust their interpretive frameworks to match these patterns, creating stability through predictability. When patterns shift, tissues must recalibrate, adjusting their responses to new temporal structures. This recalibration is not instantaneous. It unfolds over repeated exposures, reflecting the adaptive nature of interpretation.

Repeated timing patterns shape system adaptation by establishing recurring conditions that influence how signals are processed. Over time, tissues adjust their sensitivity and responsiveness to match the temporal structure of signaling. This adaptation does not change the signal itself. It changes the way the signal is interpreted. A system exposed to frequent signals may adjust by altering its responsiveness to maintain stability, while a system exposed to intermittent signals may develop a different interpretive framework. These adaptations influence routing decisions, coordination, and overall system behavior.

Adaptation to timing patterns introduces stability when patterns are coherent. Coherence allows the system to align its interpretive processes with the temporal structure of signaling, reducing variability and supporting consistent coordination. When patterns are inconsistent, adaptation becomes more complex. The system must continuously adjust to changing conditions, preventing the establishment of stable interpretive frameworks. This ongoing adjustment can lead to variability in response, as tissues interpret signals within shifting temporal contexts.

Misalignment in timing disrupts the interpretive process. When signals occur at times that conflict with established patterns or with other regulatory processes, their meaning becomes less clear. Tissues may interpret the same signal differently, leading to divergence in response. This divergence disrupts coordination, as routing decisions become inconsistent across tissues. The system must then reconcile these inconsistencies, often through compensatory adjustments that may introduce additional variability.

One form of misalignment occurs when signals overlap in ways that obscure their temporal boundaries. When signals are not clearly separated, the system may interpret them as a continuous state rather than as distinct events. This interpretation alters routing decisions, as tissues respond to what appears to be sustained availability rather than discrete inputs. Another form of misalignment involves irregular spacing, where signals do not follow a consistent pattern. This irregularity prevents the formation of stable interpretive frameworks, requiring continuous recalibration.

A further distortion arises when timing conflicts with other regulatory rhythms. The metabolic system operates within broader temporal structures that include circadian patterns and activity cycles. When insulin signaling occurs in ways that do not align with these structures, interpretation becomes more complex. Tissues must integrate conflicting temporal information, which can alter coordination and affect routing decisions. The resulting behavior reflects an attempt to reconcile competing signals within a unified response.

These distortion patterns highlight that timing is not an independent variable. It interacts with other aspects of system behavior, including coordination and interpretation. The Timing Mechanism integrates these interactions by defining how temporal placement shapes the meaning of signals within the system. It establishes that signals cannot be understood without reference to their position within sequences and that sequences cannot be understood without considering their interaction with system state and tissue-level dynamics.

The system's ability to maintain stability depends on its capacity to interpret signals within coherent temporal frameworks. When timing patterns are consistent and aligned with system conditions, interpretation supports coordinated behavior. When timing patterns are inconsistent or misaligned, interpretation becomes fragmented, leading to variability and potential instability. The Timing Mechanism provides a structure for understanding these outcomes by linking temporal placement to interpretive processes.

By emphasizing sequence over magnitude, the mechanism clarifies that the arrangement of signals across time carries more informational weight than the amplitude of individual signals in isolation. Magnitude contributes to the signal, but it is interpreted within the context of sequence. This relationship defines how the system processes information and determines its response. It also explains why identical magnitudes can produce different outcomes when their temporal placement differs.

The Timing Mechanism therefore extends the understanding of insulin beyond its role as a signal of availability. It defines how that signal is embedded within time, how it interacts with other signals, and how it is interpreted across tissues and across sequences. It establishes that timing shapes meaning, and that meaning determines coordination. Through this framework, metabolic behavior can be understood as the product of temporal organization rather than as the direct effect of isolated inputs.

In this model, stability is maintained through the alignment of timing patterns with system conditions and tissue-level responses. Signals are integrated into sequences that the system can interpret consistently, allowing for coordinated routing and allocation of energy. Disruptions to this temporal structure introduce variability, requiring adaptation or compensation. The Timing Mechanism captures these dynamics, providing a framework for understanding how temporal placement governs the interpretation and coordination of insulin signaling within the metabolic system.

The Glucose Regulation Mechanism

The Glucose Regulation Mechanism defines how circulating glucose levels are maintained within a functional range through continuous interaction between glucose availability and insulin signaling. This process is not governed by isolated events or singular responses. It operates as an ongoing regulatory loop in which glucose and insulin influence each other across time, shaping system behavior through repeated cycles of signaling, interpretation, and adjustment. Stability within this mechanism is not achieved by fixing glucose at a constant value but by maintaining controlled variation through responsive coordination.

Insulin participates in this process as a signal that reflects and responds to changes in circulating glucose. When glucose levels shift, insulin signaling adjusts in relation to those changes, communicating information about current availability to tissues involved in energy distribution and use. This signaling does not directly impose correction. It modifies the interpretive environment across tissues, influencing how glucose is handled through coordinated responses. The outcome is a dynamic balance in which glucose levels are regulated through distributed interpretation rather than centralized control.

The relationship between glucose and insulin is bidirectional. Glucose influences insulin signaling by altering the conditions under which signals are generated. As circulating glucose changes, the signaling system adjusts its output, producing patterns that correspond to the current state of availability. Insulin, in turn, influences glucose dynamics by modifying how tissues interpret and respond to that availability. This interaction creates a feedback loop in which each component continuously affects the other, producing regulation through ongoing exchange rather than discrete correction.

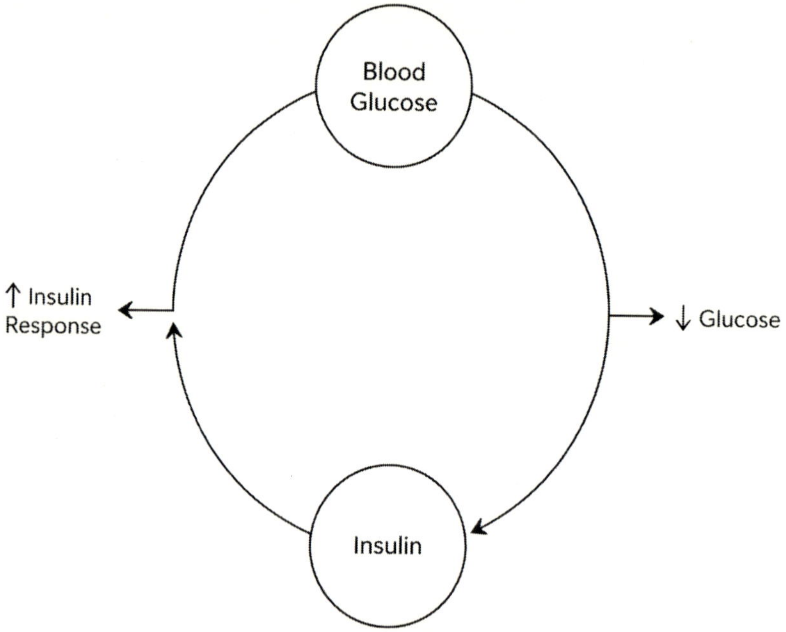

[Figure 1: Glucose–Insulin Feedback Loop]

This feedback loop operates across time as a sequence of interconnected events rather than as a single adjustment. A change in glucose initiates a signaling response that influences tissue behavior. The resulting changes in tissue-level handling of glucose alter circulating levels, which then feed back into the signaling system, modifying subsequent responses. Each cycle contributes to the overall pattern of regulation, with timing, sequence, and magnitude interacting to shape system behavior. The loop is therefore temporal in structure, extending beyond immediate reactions to include the accumulation of prior states.

Controlled regulation emerges when this loop maintains coherence across its components. Signals are generated in alignment with changes in glucose, tissues interpret these signals within consistent frameworks, and responses produce adjustments that support stability. Variation in glucose levels occurs within a range that the system can manage, with feedback operating efficiently to prevent excessive deviation. This form of regulation is characterized by responsiveness that is proportionate to conditions, allowing the system to adapt without generating instability.

Unstable or oscillatory regulation arises when coherence within the feedback loop is disrupted. This disruption can take multiple forms. Signals may be delayed relative to changes in glucose, reducing the system's ability to respond in a timely manner. Responses may be exaggerated, producing corrections that overshoot the required adjustment. Feedback may become uncoupled, with changes in glucose failing to produce appropriate signaling responses or with signaling failing to influence tissue behavior effectively. These disruptions alter the structure of the loop, leading to variability that extends beyond controlled ranges.

Timing plays a critical role in determining whether regulation remains controlled or becomes unstable. The interval between changes in glucose and corresponding adjustments in insulin signaling influences how effectively the system can respond. When timing is aligned, signals are integrated into the feedback loop in a manner that supports continuity. When timing is misaligned, signals may arrive too early, too late, or in patterns that conflict with ongoing processes. These temporal mismatches alter interpretation across tissues, affecting how glucose is handled and contributing to instability.

Coordination across tissues is also essential within the Glucose Regulation Mechanism. The liver, muscle, and adipose tissue each participate in the handling of glucose, interpreting insulin signaling within their respective roles. The liver regulates the release and retention of glucose, adjusting its behavior based on both circulating levels and signaling inputs. Muscle tissue contributes through uptake and utilization, responding to insulin in ways that reflect its energetic demands. Adipose tissue participates by adjusting its interactions with circulating substrates, contributing to the buffering of availability. The integration of these responses determines how glucose levels evolve within the system.

Interpretation links these tissue-level responses to the feedback loop. Each tissue does not respond to glucose or insulin in isolation. It integrates both within a broader signaling context that includes prior exposure, current demand, and concurrent signals. This integration determines how each tissue contributes to regulation at any given moment. When interpretation is aligned across tissues, coordination supports stable regulation. When interpretation diverges, responses may conflict, altering the trajectory of glucose levels and disrupting the feedback loop.

The Glucose Regulation Mechanism therefore operates as an integrated system in which timing, coordination, and interpretation converge. Signals are generated in response to changes in glucose, interpreted across tissues within context, and translated into coordinated actions that modify circulating levels. These actions feed back into the system, influencing subsequent signaling and interpretation. The loop continues, with each cycle shaped by the cumulative effects of prior interactions.

Adaptation occurs within this mechanism as repeated signaling patterns influence how the system processes information. Over time, tissues adjust their interpretive frameworks in response to recurring conditions. These adjustments alter sensitivity, responsiveness, and coordination, affecting how glucose regulation unfolds. A system exposed to consistent patterns may develop stable responses that support controlled regulation. A system exposed to variable or inconsistent patterns may exhibit increased variability, reflecting the absence of a coherent interpretive framework.

Adaptation does not eliminate variability. It shapes the boundaries within which variability occurs. Controlled regulation is characterized by fluctuations that remain within a range that the system can manage. Unstable regulation involves fluctuations that exceed this range, often as a result of misaligned timing, disrupted coordination, or altered interpretation. The distinction between these states is not based on the presence or absence of change but on the structure of the feedback loop and its ability to integrate signals effectively.

Failure patterns within the Glucose Regulation Mechanism reflect disruptions to the feedback loop. Delayed signaling reduces the system's ability to respond to changes in glucose, allowing deviations to persist longer than intended. Exaggerated responses introduce instability by producing corrections that overshoot, creating oscillations as the system attempts to re-establish balance. Uncoupled feedback occurs when signaling and response become disconnected, with changes in glucose failing to produce appropriate adjustments or with adjustments failing to influence glucose effectively.

These failure patterns often interact. Delays can lead to exaggerated responses as the system compensates for accumulated deviation. Exaggeration can create oscillatory behavior, where corrections alternate between overshoot and undershoot. Uncoupling can amplify both effects by reducing the system's ability to integrate signals and responses coherently. The resulting behavior reflects a breakdown in the regulatory loop rather than a failure of any single component.

The role of insulin within this mechanism remains consistent across these conditions. It functions as a signal that participates in the feedback loop, communicating information about glucose availability and influencing tissue responses. Its effectiveness depends on how it is integrated within the loop. When timing, coordination, and interpretation are aligned, insulin contributes to stable regulation. When these elements are disrupted, the same signal may produce outcomes that do not support stability, reflecting changes in the system rather than changes in the signal itself.

The Glucose Regulation Mechanism demonstrates that stability is an emergent property of interaction rather than a fixed outcome. It arises from the continuous exchange between glucose and insulin, mediated by tissue-level responses and shaped by temporal dynamics. The system does not maintain stability by preventing change. It maintains stability by managing change through responsive signaling and coordinated interpretation.

This framework clarifies that glucose regulation cannot be understood through static measurements or isolated variables. It requires analysis of how signals interact across time, how tissues coordinate their responses, and how interpretation evolves based on prior exposure. The feedback loop provides the structure through which these elements interact, defining how the system adapts to changing conditions while maintaining functional balance.

By situating insulin within this loop, the mechanism emphasizes its role as part of a dynamic regulatory process. It is not a force that acts independently on glucose levels. It is a signal that participates in a continuous exchange, shaping and being shaped by the conditions it reflects. The stability of glucose levels depends on the integrity of this exchange, on the alignment of timing and coordination, and on the capacity of the system to interpret signals within context.

The Glucose Regulation Mechanism therefore integrates signaling, interpretation, and response into a unified model of metabolic regulation. It establishes that control is achieved through feedback that operates across time, through coordination that emerges from distributed interpretation, and through adaptation that shapes how signals are processed. Instability arises when this integration is disrupted, altering the structure of the loop and the behavior it produces.

Within this model, glucose levels are not controlled by direct intervention but by the ongoing interaction between signals and responses. Insulin contributes to this interaction by conveying information about availability, influencing how tissues handle glucose, and participating in the feedback that defines regulation. The system's ability to maintain stability depends on how effectively this interaction is maintained, demonstrating that regulation is a continuous process shaped by the dynamics of signaling rather than by isolated events.

The Energy Partitioning Mechanism

The Energy Partitioning Mechanism defines how available energy is allocated across competing pathways of immediate use, circulation, and storage through coordinated interpretation of insulin signaling and related inputs. It does not describe a fixed distribution rule or a static preference for one pathway over another. It describes a dynamic process in which allocation decisions are made continuously, shaped by current demand, prior conditions, and the signaling environment within which those decisions are interpreted. Partitioning is not an outcome applied after energy appears in circulation. It is the process through which energy is directed as it moves through the system.

Energy entering circulation represents potential rather than destination. It is not inherently assigned to use or storage. The system evaluates this availability in relation to its current state, determining how energy should be routed to maintain stability. Insulin participates in this evaluation by signaling the presence and pattern of availability, but it does not impose a singular pathway. It modifies the informational context within which tissues interpret how to allocate resources. The result is a coordinated distribution that reflects both the signal and the system interpreting it.

Allocation occurs across three primary domains: immediate use within active tissues, continued circulation for redistribution, and storage for deferred use. These domains are not independent compartments. They are interconnected pathways through which energy flows, with transitions occurring continuously based on system conditions. The Energy Partitioning Mechanism describes how the system determines the proportion of energy directed toward each domain at any given moment, balancing present requirements with future stability.

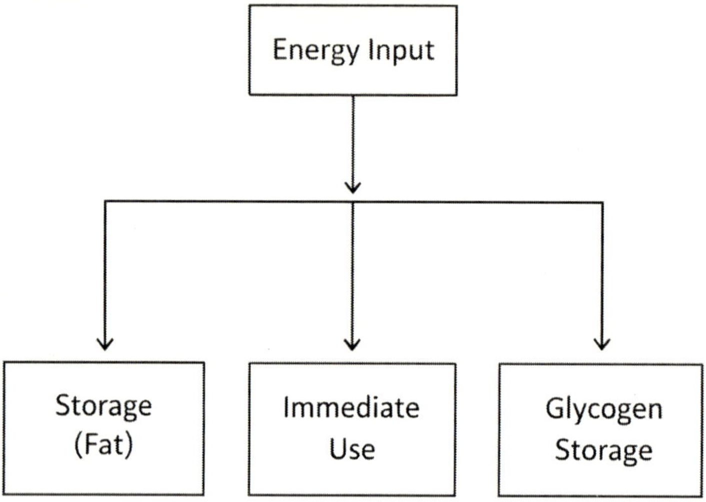

[Figure 2: Energy Partitioning Pathways]

Immediate use reflects the system's capacity to direct energy toward active processes. This pathway is influenced by tissue demand, particularly within muscle, where uptake and utilization are aligned with current activity and internal requirements. Circulation represents the maintenance of availability across the system, allowing energy to remain accessible for redistribution. Storage reflects the allocation of energy to buffering domains, primarily within adipose tissue, where it can be retained for future use. The system continuously adjusts the balance between these pathways, ensuring that energy is neither insufficiently available nor excessively accumulated in a manner that disrupts coordination.

Insulin influences partitioning by shaping how tissues interpret the presence of circulating energy. It communicates that energy is available for distribution, altering the probabilities associated with different allocation pathways. This influence is not uniform across tissues. Muscle, liver, and adipose tissue each integrate insulin signaling within their own functional context, contributing to partitioning through distributed interpretation. Muscle may increase uptake for immediate use when demand is elevated. The liver may adjust its regulation of circulating substrates, influencing the availability of energy for redistribution. Adipose tissue may modify its buffering behavior, contributing to storage when conditions support deferred allocation.

Priority pathways emerge from the interaction between signaling and system conditions. Under conditions of elevated demand, allocation may favor immediate use, directing energy toward tissues capable of utilizing it efficiently. Under conditions of relative surplus, allocation may shift toward storage, buffering energy to maintain stability over time. When circulation requires maintenance, the system may preserve availability, delaying allocation until conditions clarify. These priority pathways are not predetermined. They are determined continuously through interpretation, reflecting the current balance of demand, availability, and prior state.

Prior state plays a critical role in shaping partitioning decisions. The system does not evaluate each instance of energy availability in isolation. It integrates current signals with the history of prior allocation patterns, adjusting its behavior based on accumulated conditions. A system that has recently directed substantial energy toward storage may interpret subsequent signals differently than a system that has prioritized immediate use. These differences influence how energy is partitioned, demonstrating that allocation is conditioned by both present inputs and past behavior.

Coordination across tissues is required for partitioning to function effectively. Each tissue contributes to allocation through its interpretation of signaling, but these contributions must align within a shared framework. The liver influences the availability of substrates entering circulation, shaping the pool from which allocation occurs. Muscle determines how much energy is directed toward immediate use, influencing overall demand. Adipose tissue modulates buffering, affecting how much energy is retained for future use. The integration of these roles produces the partitioning pattern observed at the system level.

The Energy Partitioning Mechanism therefore depends on coherence across tissues. When interpretations align, allocation supports stability, with energy directed toward pathways that match system requirements. When interpretations diverge, allocation becomes fragmented, with energy routed inconsistently across domains. This fragmentation disrupts coordination, producing imbalances that affect both immediate function and long-term stability. Partitioning is thus an expression of coordinated interpretation rather than an isolated process.

Adaptive allocation reflects the system's ability to adjust partitioning in response to changing conditions. In this state, routing decisions are responsive to signals, with energy directed according to current demand and availability. The system remains flexible, adjusting allocation as conditions evolve. Persistent allocation reflects a different state, in which routing patterns become fixed or biased, continuing even when conditions change. In this state, partitioning no longer reflects current signals accurately. It reflects the inertia of prior patterns, reducing the system's ability to adapt.

The distinction between adaptive and persistent allocation is not defined by the presence of a particular pathway but by the responsiveness of the system to signaling. Adaptive systems shift allocation as conditions change, maintaining alignment between signals and outcomes. Persistent systems maintain allocation patterns despite changes in signaling, producing outcomes that may not support stability. This persistence can arise from repeated exposure to consistent signaling patterns, which shape interpretation in ways that become resistant to change.

Repeated signaling patterns influence partitioning by establishing expectations within the system. When signals occur in consistent sequences, tissues adjust their interpretive frameworks to match these patterns, producing predictable allocation responses. Over time, these responses become embedded within system behavior, influencing how new signals are interpreted. When patterns change, the system must adapt, recalibrating its interpretive frameworks to align with new conditions. The speed and completeness of this adaptation determine whether partitioning remains adaptive or becomes persistent.

Timing, coordination, and interpretation converge within partitioning behavior. Timing determines when signals are received and how they relate to prior sequences. Coordination ensures that tissues align their responses within a shared framework. Interpretation translates signals into allocation decisions within each tissue. Together, these elements define how energy is partitioned across domains, producing outcomes that reflect the integrated behavior of the system. Partitioning is therefore not a single mechanism but the expression of multiple mechanisms operating in concert.

Observable metabolic outcomes emerge from partitioning patterns. The distribution of energy across use, circulation, and storage determines how the system functions at both immediate and extended time scales. When partitioning aligns with demand and availability, outcomes reflect stability, with energy supporting both current activity and future needs. When partitioning becomes biased or misaligned, outcomes reflect imbalance, with energy accumulating or depleting in ways that disrupt coordination. These outcomes are not direct effects of signals but the result of how signals are interpreted and translated into allocation.

Failure patterns within the Energy Partitioning Mechanism arise when allocation becomes rigid, biased, or disconnected from current conditions. Rigidity occurs when partitioning patterns persist despite changes in signaling, reducing the system's ability to adjust. Bias emerges when allocation consistently favors one pathway over others, regardless of demand or availability. Misalignment occurs when tissues interpret signals differently, producing conflicting routing decisions that disrupt coordination. Each of these patterns reflects a breakdown in the adaptive process that defines effective partitioning.

Rigid partitioning limits the system's capacity to respond to variability. When allocation patterns become fixed, the system cannot adjust routing in response to changing conditions. This limitation can produce accumulation in storage pathways or insufficient allocation to immediate use, depending on the direction of the bias. Biased partitioning further distorts allocation by consistently directing energy toward specific pathways, reducing flexibility and increasing the likelihood of imbalance. Misaligned partitioning introduces inconsistency, with different tissues contributing to allocation in ways that do not align, producing variability that the system must reconcile.

These failure patterns are often reinforced over time through repeated signaling. Persistent exposure to specific patterns can entrench interpretive frameworks that support rigidity or bias. As these frameworks become more established, the system's ability to adapt decreases, and partitioning becomes increasingly disconnected from current conditions. The resulting instability reflects not a failure of the signals themselves but a failure of interpretation and coordination within the system.

The Energy Partitioning Mechanism demonstrates that metabolic outcomes are determined by how energy is allocated rather than by the presence of energy alone. Insulin contributes to this allocation by providing information about availability, influencing how tissues interpret and respond to that availability. Its role is not to direct energy into specific pathways but to shape the context within which routing decisions are made. The resulting partitioning reflects the integrated behavior of the system, influenced by timing, coordination, and interpretation across tissues.

Within this framework, stability is maintained through adaptive partitioning that aligns with current conditions. The system continuously adjusts allocation to balance immediate use, circulation, and storage, ensuring that energy supports both present function and future needs. Instability arises when this adjustment process is disrupted, leading to partitioning patterns that no longer reflect the system's requirements. The Energy Partitioning Mechanism captures these dynamics, providing a structure for understanding how energy distribution shapes metabolic behavior over time.

By defining partitioning as a dynamic, signal-based process, the mechanism clarifies that allocation is not predetermined or static. It is the outcome of continuous interaction between signals, tissues, and conditions, evolving as the system adapts to variability. This perspective allows for a more precise understanding of how metabolic stability is maintained and how deviations from adaptive partitioning contribute to instability.

The Clearance Mechanism

The Clearance Mechanism defines how insulin signaling is brought to resolution through the progressive removal of the signal from circulation and the corresponding reduction of its interpretive influence across tissues. It establishes the boundary conditions of signaling by determining how long a signal remains active within the system and how it transitions back toward baseline. This process is not an afterthought to signaling. It is integral to how signaling is structured, interpreted, and integrated into broader metabolic behavior. Without clearance, signals would not have definable duration, and without definable duration, interpretation would lose temporal specificity.

Insulin signaling begins with the introduction of a signal that communicates energy availability. It does not end at peak concentration. The decline of that signal is equally significant, as it defines the period during which tissues continue to interpret and respond to its presence. Clearance governs this decline. It determines how quickly the signal is reduced, how sharply it resolves, and how clearly the system transitions from one interpretive state to another. The mechanism therefore establishes that signal duration, not magnitude alone, defines the informational structure of insulin signaling.

The return toward baseline is not a passive disappearance of signal. It is an active process involving multiple tissues, with the liver occupying a central role. As insulin circulates, it is progressively removed through hepatic processing and through uptake and degradation in peripheral tissues. This removal reduces the concentration of the signal, but more importantly, it alters the interpretive environment across the system. As levels decline, tissues adjust their responses, shifting from states associated with availability toward states that reflect reduced signaling presence. The trajectory of this decline shapes how these transitions occur.

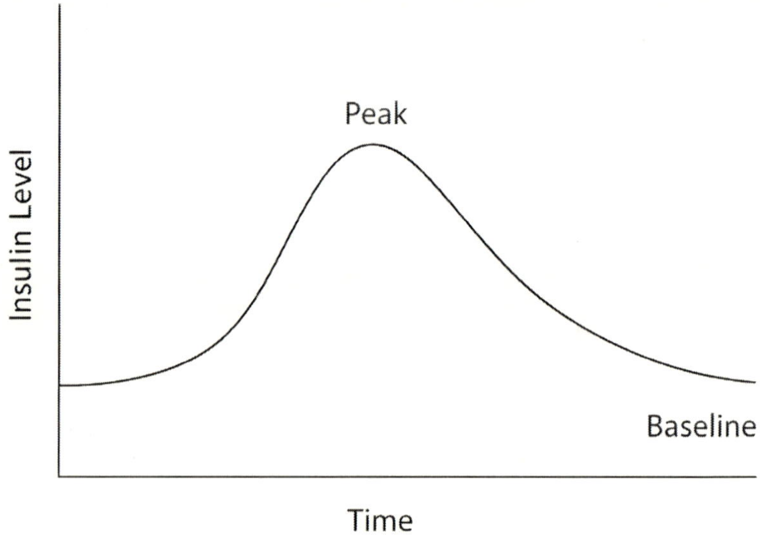

[Figure 3: Insulin Clearance Curve]

The Clearance Mechanism is therefore defined by the curve of signal reduction rather than by a singular endpoint. The slope, duration, and continuity of this curve determine how the signal is experienced by the system. A rapid decline produces a clear boundary between signaling states, allowing tissues to distinguish between periods of active signaling and periods of relative absence. A prolonged decline extends the period of interpretive influence, blurring these boundaries and altering how subsequent signals are integrated. The curve becomes the temporal structure through which the signal is understood.

The liver plays a central role in shaping this structure by acting as a primary site of insulin clearance. It does not merely remove insulin as a substance. It participates in defining the duration of the signal as it is interpreted across the system. By modulating how quickly insulin is reduced in circulation, the liver influences how long tissues remain within a given interpretive state. Peripheral tissues contribute to this process as well, participating in uptake and degradation that further shapes the clearance profile. The combined effect of these processes determines the overall duration of signaling.

Duration influences interpretation because tissues do not respond to instantaneous levels alone. They respond to the persistence of a signal over time. A signal that rises and falls rapidly is interpreted differently than a signal that remains elevated for an extended period, even if peak levels are similar. Persistence conveys information about the continuity of availability, shaping how tissues coordinate their responses. Prolonged duration may be interpreted as sustained availability, leading to allocation patterns that differ from those associated with transient signals. The meaning of the signal is therefore encoded in its duration as much as in its magnitude.

This temporal encoding interacts with coordination across tissues. Muscle, liver, and adipose tissue interpret signal duration within their respective roles, adjusting their behavior based on how long the signal persists. Muscle tissue may extend its period of uptake and utilization when signaling is prolonged, altering the balance between immediate use and other pathways. The liver may adjust its regulation of circulating substrates over a longer interval, affecting how energy is distributed across the system. Adipose tissue may modify its buffering behavior in response to sustained signaling, influencing storage dynamics. These adjustments occur in parallel, producing coordinated outcomes that reflect the duration of the signal.

Timing is inseparable from clearance. The placement of a signal within a sequence depends not only on when it begins but on when it ends. Clearance defines this endpoint, determining how signals overlap, how they are spaced, and how they interact across time. When clearance is rapid, signals remain distinct, allowing the system to interpret sequences with clarity. When clearance is delayed, signals may overlap, creating composite patterns that alter interpretation. The interaction between timing and clearance therefore shapes the structure of signaling sequences and the meaning derived from them.

Prolonged signaling alters coordination, timing, and partitioning simultaneously. Extended duration increases the likelihood of overlap between signals, modifying how sequences are constructed. It extends the interpretive influence of each signal, affecting how tissues coordinate their responses. It shifts partitioning by maintaining conditions associated with availability for longer periods, influencing how energy is allocated across pathways. These changes are not independent. They interact, producing system-level effects that reflect the combined influence of extended signal duration.

The Clearance Mechanism also integrates with feedback regulation. As insulin signaling influences glucose dynamics and other aspects of metabolic behavior, the duration of that signaling affects how feedback loops operate. Prolonged signals extend the period during which feedback is active, potentially altering the timing and magnitude of subsequent responses. Rapid clearance shortens this period, creating more discrete cycles of feedback. The structure of these cycles influences how effectively the system maintains stability, demonstrating that clearance is a critical component of feedback regulation.

Over time, repeated patterns of clearance shape system adaptation. Consistent patterns of rapid resolution may lead to interpretive frameworks that emphasize discrete signaling events, with tissues adjusting their responsiveness to match these patterns. Repeated patterns of delayed clearance may lead to frameworks that interpret signals as more continuous, altering sensitivity and coordination. These adaptations influence how future signals are processed, demonstrating that clearance patterns contribute to the development of system behavior over time.

Adaptation to clearance patterns is not uniform across tissues. Each tissue integrates duration within its own context, adjusting its interpretive processes accordingly. These adjustments influence how coordination emerges, as tissues align their responses based on shared exposure to clearance patterns. When patterns are consistent, coordination may stabilize around predictable responses. When patterns are inconsistent, tissues may adapt differently, introducing variability into coordination and affecting overall system behavior.

Failure patterns within the Clearance Mechanism arise when the termination of signaling becomes impaired, delayed, or inconsistent. Impaired clearance reduces the system's ability to resolve signals effectively, extending duration beyond what is aligned with current conditions. Delayed clearance alters the temporal structure of signaling sequences, increasing overlap and reducing clarity in interpretation. Inconsistent clearance introduces variability, preventing the system from establishing stable interpretive frameworks. Each of these patterns disrupts the boundaries that define signaling states, affecting coordination and partitioning.

Delayed clearance can lead to sustained interpretive states that do not match actual conditions. When signals persist beyond the period of availability they represent, tissues may continue to respond as if conditions have not changed. This persistence alters allocation patterns, potentially directing energy in ways that do not support stability. Impaired clearance can amplify this effect by further extending duration, increasing the divergence between signaling and underlying conditions. The resulting behavior reflects a mismatch between information and interpretation.

Inconsistent clearance introduces additional complexity. When the duration of signals varies unpredictably, the system cannot rely on stable temporal patterns to guide interpretation. Tissues must continuously adjust to changing durations, preventing the formation of consistent coordination. This variability can produce fluctuations in partitioning and feedback regulation, as each signal is interpreted within a different temporal context. The system remains responsive but lacks the coherence required for stable behavior.

These failure patterns highlight that clearance is not a secondary feature of signaling. It is a defining component of how signals are structured and understood. The ability of the system to maintain stability depends on its capacity to resolve signals in a manner that aligns with current conditions and supports coherent interpretation across tissues. When clearance functions effectively, it creates clear boundaries between signaling states, allowing the system to transition smoothly between conditions. When it is disrupted, these boundaries become blurred, altering how signals are integrated and how responses are coordinated.

The Clearance Mechanism therefore establishes that signal duration is a primary determinant of meaning within the metabolic system. Insulin operates as information that unfolds across time, and clearance defines the endpoint of that unfolding. By shaping how long the signal persists, the mechanism influences interpretation, coordination, and partitioning, integrating these processes into a unified temporal structure. Stability emerges when this structure remains aligned with system conditions, allowing signals to be interpreted accurately and responses to be coordinated effectively.

Within this framework, insulin is not defined by its peak presence but by its temporal profile. The rise and fall of the signal, governed by clearance, determine how it is experienced by the system and how it contributes to ongoing regulation. The Clearance Mechanism provides the structure through which this profile is understood, emphasizing that the boundaries of signaling are as significant as the signals themselves in determining metabolic behavior.

The Sensitivity Mechanism

The Sensitivity Mechanism defines how insulin signaling is translated into action through the responsiveness of tissues and cells to that signal. It establishes that the presence of a signal does not determine its effect independently. The effect emerges through the capacity of the system to receive, interpret, and act on that signal. Sensitivity therefore operates as the interface between signaling and response, shaping how informational input is converted into coordinated metabolic behavior. Without sensitivity, signaling would not produce structured outcomes. Without variability in sensitivity, the system would lack the capacity to adjust its responses to changing conditions. Sensitivity, in this context, is the degree to which a given insulin signal is translated into coordinated action across tissues based on current responsiveness, prior exposure, and system state.

Sensitivity is not a static property. It reflects the current state of tissues, their recent exposure to signaling patterns, and the broader context within which signals are interpreted. Cells do not respond uniformly to insulin. They exhibit varying degrees of responsiveness that influence how strongly and how efficiently signals are translated into action. This variation is not random. It is structured by both intrinsic characteristics of the tissue and by the history of signaling that has shaped its interpretive framework.

The distinction between efficient signaling and impaired response emerges within this context. Efficient signaling occurs when the informational content of insulin is translated into coordinated action with minimal distortion. Tissues interpret the signal in alignment with current conditions, producing responses that support stability across the system. Impaired response occurs when this translation is altered, delayed, or diminished, leading to outcomes that do not fully reflect the informational content of the signal. The signal remains present, but its meaning is not expressed accurately in the resulting behavior.

Sensitivity determines how signals are weighted within the interpretive process. A signal of a given magnitude and duration may produce a strong response in one tissue and a limited response in another, depending on their respective sensitivities. This weighting influences how coordination emerges, as tissues contribute to system behavior based on their responsiveness. Sensitivity therefore acts as a scaling factor within the broader signaling framework, modifying how information is distributed and acted upon across the system.

Sensitivity operates across a gradient rather than as a binary state of responsiveness. Tissues do not shift between fully responsive and fully impaired conditions. They adjust continuously, expressing varying degrees of responsiveness that influence how signals are interpreted and acted upon. This gradient introduces nuance into the signaling system, as changes in sensitivity alter not only the strength of response but the meaning of the signal itself. A signal interpreted within a highly responsive context may indicate sufficient availability to support immediate allocation, while the same signal within a reduced responsiveness context may be interpreted as insufficient, requiring prolonged exposure or additional signaling to produce a comparable effect. The informational content of the signal is therefore not fixed. It is modulated by the responsiveness of the system interpreting it, demonstrating that sensitivity shapes both the magnitude and the interpretation of signaling outcomes.

Tissue-specific variation in sensitivity is a defining feature of the mechanism. Muscle tissue, hepatic tissue, and adipose tissue each exhibit distinct patterns of responsiveness that reflect their roles within the metabolic system. Muscle tissue adjusts its responsiveness in relation to its capacity for uptake and utilization, aligning sensitivity with demand and internal state. The liver modulates its responsiveness to balance its role in maintaining circulating energy levels, integrating insulin signaling with other regulatory inputs. Adipose tissue adjusts its sensitivity in relation to its buffering function, influencing how it participates in storage and release dynamics. These variations allow the system to distribute responses in a manner that supports coordinated behavior.

The integration of these tissue-specific responses defines how sensitivity shapes overall system behavior. When sensitivities are aligned across tissues, signals are translated into coordinated actions that support stability. When sensitivities diverge, responses may become unbalanced, with some tissues responding strongly while others respond weakly or inconsistently. This divergence alters routing, partitioning, and regulation, demonstrating that sensitivity is not only a local property but a system-level determinant of behavior.

Sensitivity interacts with timing by influencing how signals are interpreted across sequences. A tissue with high responsiveness may react quickly to a signal, integrating it into ongoing sequences with minimal delay. A tissue with reduced responsiveness may require longer exposure or repeated signals to produce a comparable effect. This difference alters how signals are positioned within temporal sequences, affecting how they overlap, how they are spaced, and how they contribute to coordination. Timing and sensitivity therefore operate together to define how signals are experienced across time.

Coordination is similarly shaped by sensitivity. The distribution of responsiveness across tissues determines how signals are translated into coordinated action. When sensitivity is balanced, tissues align their responses within a shared framework, producing coherent routing and allocation. When sensitivity is uneven, coordination becomes more complex, as tissues contribute to system behavior with differing intensities and timing. This complexity can introduce variability into partitioning and regulation, requiring additional adjustments to maintain stability.

Partitioning is directly influenced by sensitivity through its effect on allocation decisions. Tissues with higher responsiveness may contribute more strongly to immediate use or storage pathways, depending on their role and the signaling context. Tissues with lower responsiveness may contribute less, altering the balance of allocation across domains. These differences shape how energy is distributed across use, circulation, and storage, demonstrating that partitioning outcomes reflect not only signaling patterns but also the responsiveness of the system interpreting those patterns.

Clearance interacts with sensitivity by defining the duration over which signals can be interpreted. A highly responsive tissue may require only brief exposure to a signal to initiate a response, while a less responsive tissue may depend on prolonged duration to achieve a similar effect. Changes in clearance therefore alter how sensitivity is expressed, as they modify the temporal window within which interpretation occurs. Prolonged signals may compensate for reduced responsiveness in some contexts, while rapid clearance may limit the impact of signals even in responsive tissues. The interaction between clearance and sensitivity shapes how signals are translated into action across time.

Sensitivity is not fixed across time. It adapts based on repeated exposure to signaling patterns. Tissues adjust their responsiveness in response to the frequency, magnitude, and duration of signals they encounter. Repeated exposure to consistent patterns may lead to adjustments that alter how future signals are interpreted. These adjustments are not uniform. They reflect the specific patterns of exposure and the functional role of each tissue. Over time, these changes influence coordination, timing, and partitioning, demonstrating that sensitivity is both a product and a determinant of system behavior.

Adaptation within the Sensitivity Mechanism reflects the system's attempt to maintain stability under changing conditions. When signaling patterns are coherent and aligned with system demands, sensitivity may adjust in ways that support efficient translation of signals into action. When patterns are inconsistent or misaligned, sensitivity may adjust in ways that reflect the need to manage variability, potentially altering responsiveness in ways that affect coordination. These adaptations influence how signals are interpreted, shaping system behavior over extended periods.

Altered sensitivity reshapes system behavior by modifying how signals are translated into coordinated responses. Changes in responsiveness can amplify or diminish the impact of signals, altering routing, partitioning, and regulation. These changes may occur gradually, reflecting cumulative adaptation, or more abruptly in response to shifts in signaling patterns or system conditions. The resulting behavior reflects the interaction between signals and the responsiveness of the system interpreting them.

Failure patterns within the Sensitivity Mechanism arise when responsiveness becomes reduced, inconsistent, or misaligned with system requirements. Reduced sensitivity limits the system's ability to translate signals into action, requiring stronger or more prolonged signals to achieve comparable responses. This limitation alters timing and coordination, as signals must persist longer to produce effects, increasing the likelihood of overlap and misalignment. Inconsistent sensitivity introduces variability, with tissues responding unpredictably to signals, disrupting coordination and partitioning.

Misaligned sensitivity occurs when responsiveness does not reflect current conditions or system demands. In this state, tissues may respond strongly when reduced responsiveness would support stability or respond weakly when stronger responses are required. This misalignment disrupts the balance of allocation and regulation, producing outcomes that do not support system stability. These failure patterns are not caused by changes in the signal itself but by changes in how the signal is interpreted and acted upon.

These patterns often interact with other mechanisms, amplifying their effects. Reduced sensitivity may contribute to prolonged signaling as the system attempts to compensate, altering clearance dynamics. Inconsistent sensitivity may disrupt timing sequences, affecting how signals are integrated across time. Misaligned sensitivity may distort partitioning, directing energy in ways that do not match system conditions. The Sensitivity Mechanism therefore operates within a network of interactions, influencing and being influenced by other aspects of system behavior.

The Sensitivity Mechanism establishes that the effectiveness of insulin signaling is not determined by the signal alone. It is determined by the responsiveness of the system receiving that signal. Sensitivity defines how information is translated into action, shaping how coordination emerges, how timing is structured, and how energy is partitioned. It provides the link between signaling and outcome, demonstrating that metabolic behavior reflects not only the presence of signals but the capacity of the system to respond to them.

Within this framework, stability is maintained when sensitivity supports accurate and efficient translation of signals into coordinated responses. Instability arises when responsiveness is altered in ways that disrupt this translation, leading to variability and misalignment across tissues and processes. The Sensitivity Mechanism captures these dynamics, emphasizing that responsiveness is a central determinant of how signaling patterns influence system behavior over time.

The Resistance Mechanism

The Resistance Mechanism defines how insulin signaling loses clarity and effectiveness as it is translated into coordinated metabolic response. It does not describe the absence of signaling, nor does it imply that the signal ceases to exist. It describes a condition in which the signal remains present but its informational content is no longer interpreted or expressed with the same precision or consistency. Resistance therefore operates as a degradation of signal fidelity, altering how information is transmitted through the system and how that information is converted into action across tissues. Resistance, in this context, is the progressive reduction in the clarity and effectiveness with which insulin signaling is translated into coordinated metabolic response across tissues.

Signal clarity depends on the alignment between input and response. When insulin signaling is interpreted accurately, tissues respond in ways that reflect the information conveyed, producing coordinated behavior that supports stability. Resistance emerges when this alignment begins to shift. The signal continues to circulate, but its meaning becomes less distinct within the interpretive framework of the system. Responses may become diminished, delayed, or altered in direction, reflecting a breakdown in the translation process rather than a disappearance of the signal itself.

This distinction separates resistance from absence. In the absence of signaling, there is no informational input to interpret. In resistance, the input remains, but its transmission is distorted. The system receives the signal but does not express it effectively in coordinated behavior. This creates a condition in which signaling and response are no longer tightly coupled, introducing variability into metabolic processes that depend on their alignment.

As resistance progresses, the informational content of insulin signaling becomes increasingly distorted rather than simply weakened. The signal is not only reduced in its ability to produce response, but altered in the way it is interpreted within the system. A signal that would previously indicate sufficient availability to support coordinated allocation may, under conditions of resistance, be interpreted as insufficient or ambiguous. This distortion changes how tissues prioritize pathways, how they coordinate responses, and how they integrate signals across time. The effect is not a simple reduction in output but a transformation in the meaning of the signal itself, demonstrating that resistance modifies interpretation as well as response.

Resistance is not a binary state that appears abruptly. It develops progressively as patterns of signaling and interpretation shift over time. Early in this process, changes may be subtle, with minor reductions in responsiveness or slight alterations in timing. As the process continues, these changes accumulate, producing more pronounced divergence between signal and response. The system does not transition from full sensitivity to complete resistance in a single step. It moves along a continuum in which the fidelity of signaling gradually declines.

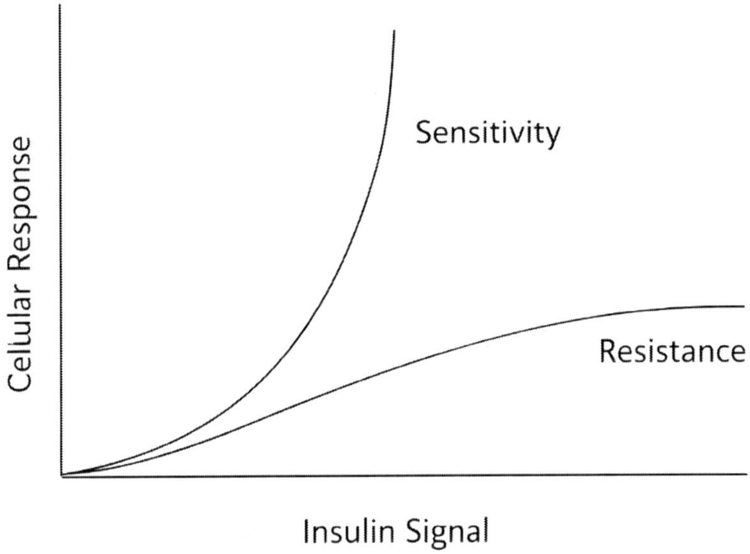

[Figure 4: Sensitivity vs Resistance Curve]

This continuum reflects the relationship between sensitivity and resistance as interdependent expressions of the same underlying process. Sensitivity defines the capacity of tissues to translate signals into coordinated action. Resistance defines the degree to which this capacity is reduced or distorted. They are not opposing categories but points along a spectrum of responsiveness. As sensitivity declines, resistance increases, not as a separate state but as a manifestation of altered signal interpretation.

The progression of resistance is shaped by repeated signaling patterns and the system's adaptation to those patterns. Signals do not act in isolation. They are experienced as sequences over time, and these sequences influence how tissues adjust their interpretive frameworks. When patterns of signaling are consistent, tissues adapt to those patterns, modifying their responsiveness to maintain stability under those conditions. This adaptation can alter how future signals are interpreted, particularly when patterns involve sustained or repeated exposure that reshapes the system's expectations.

As adaptation occurs, the meaning of signals can shift. A signal that previously conveyed a clear indication of availability may become less distinct when experienced within a different pattern of exposure. The system may adjust its responsiveness to manage perceived continuity in signaling, altering how strongly or how quickly it responds. This adjustment reflects an attempt to stabilize behavior under new conditions, but it also introduces distortion into the relationship between signal and response.

Resistance therefore emerges not as a malfunction but as a consequence of adaptation under specific signaling conditions. The system adjusts its interpretive processes to maintain stability within the context it experiences. When that context involves patterns that reduce the need for strong or immediate responses, sensitivity may decline as part of this adjustment. The resulting resistance reflects a shift in how signals are processed rather than a failure of the signaling system itself.

This shift alters interpretation across tissues. Muscle, liver, and adipose tissue may each adjust their responsiveness in ways that reflect their roles and exposure patterns. These adjustments are not necessarily uniform, leading to variation in how signals are translated into action across tissues. Divergence in responsiveness affects coordination, as tissues contribute to system behavior with differing intensities and timing. The resulting pattern reflects a system in which the signal is no longer interpreted consistently across its components.

Timing is affected as resistance progresses. Reduced responsiveness may delay the translation of signals into action, extending the interval between signal reception and response. This delay alters the temporal structure of signaling sequences, increasing the likelihood of overlap between signals and reducing the clarity of their boundaries. As timing becomes less precise, coordination across tissues becomes more complex, with responses occurring at different points within the sequence rather than in aligned patterns.

Partitioning is similarly reshaped by resistance. As responsiveness changes, the allocation of energy across pathways is influenced by altered interpretation of signaling. Tissues that respond less strongly may contribute less to immediate use or storage, shifting the balance of allocation across domains. These shifts are not necessarily uniform or predictable, as they depend on how each tissue's responsiveness has been altered. The resulting partitioning patterns reflect the cumulative effect of changes in sensitivity across the system.

The integration of resistance with sensitivity as a continuum clarifies that both mechanisms describe the same underlying process from different perspectives. Sensitivity emphasizes the capacity for accurate translation of signals into action. Resistance emphasizes the degradation of that capacity. Together, they describe how the system modulates its responsiveness over time, shaping how signaling patterns influence behavior. This integration allows for a more precise understanding of how metabolic dynamics evolve as responsiveness changes.

Feedback regulation is affected by resistance through its impact on the coupling between signal and response. When responses are diminished or delayed, the feedback loop that relies on these responses becomes altered. Changes in glucose dynamics may not produce proportional adjustments in signaling, or signaling may not produce proportional adjustments in tissue behavior. This decoupling introduces variability into the feedback process, affecting how effectively the system can maintain stability across cycles of regulation.

As resistance progresses, feedback loops may exhibit altered dynamics. Delays in response can lead to extended deviations before correction occurs. Diminished responses may require repeated or prolonged signaling to achieve adjustment, altering the structure of the loop. These changes affect how the system processes information over time, influencing both immediate regulation and longer-term adaptation. The feedback loop remains active, but its behavior reflects the altered relationship between signal and response.

System behavior is reshaped as resistance influences coordination, timing, and partitioning simultaneously. The combined effect of these changes produces patterns of variability that differ from those observed under conditions of higher sensitivity. These patterns are not random. They reflect the system's attempt to operate within a framework of altered responsiveness, integrating signals in ways that reflect its current interpretive capacity. The resulting behavior may maintain a degree of stability, but it does so under different constraints and with different dynamics.

Failure patterns within the Resistance Mechanism are best understood as progressive degradation of signal-response alignment. Early in this process, the system may compensate for minor distortions through adjustments in timing or allocation. As degradation increases, these compensatory mechanisms may become less effective, leading to more pronounced divergence between signaling and response. This divergence manifests as variability in coordination, inconsistencies in partitioning, and alterations in feedback regulation.

The degradation is cumulative. Each shift in responsiveness influences subsequent interpretation, creating a trajectory in which the system moves further from its original alignment. This trajectory is shaped by ongoing exposure to signaling patterns and the system's adaptation to those patterns. It does not follow a fixed path, but it reflects the interaction between signals, interpretation, and response over time.

The Resistance Mechanism therefore defines resistance as a process of signal degradation within the metabolic system. It emphasizes that signals can remain present while their meaning becomes less distinct, altering how they are translated into coordinated action. By framing resistance as a progressive distortion rather than a binary state, the mechanism captures the dynamic nature of responsiveness and its influence on system behavior.

Within this framework, insulin remains a signal that communicates energy availability. Its role does not change as resistance develops. What changes is the system's capacity to interpret and act on that signal with clarity and precision. The resulting behavior reflects the interaction between signaling patterns and the evolving responsiveness of the system, demonstrating that metabolic stability and instability emerge from the quality of signal interpretation rather than from the presence of signals alone.

The Compensation Mechanism

The Compensation Mechanism defines how the metabolic system increases signaling output to preserve functional alignment when responsiveness to insulin becomes reduced. It operates within the signaling layer as an adaptive response to altered interpretation, maintaining coordination by amplifying the informational signal in an attempt to preserve its effective transmission. Compensation does not restore the original interpretive state. It modifies the signaling environment to achieve comparable outcomes under changed conditions, extending the system's capacity to maintain apparent stability despite underlying distortion.

This mechanism emerges when sensitivity declines along the continuum described in the preceding framework. As tissues translate insulin signaling less effectively into coordinated action, the relationship between signal and response becomes attenuated. The system detects this attenuation through feedback processes that monitor the alignment between expected and actual outcomes. In response, signaling output increases, not as an independent escalation but as an attempt to re-establish sufficient informational influence to produce coordinated responses. The signal is not replaced. It is intensified in order to maintain its functional effect.

Compensation reframes the relationship between signal strength and system stability. Stability is not preserved by maintaining consistent signaling levels, but by maintaining sufficient signal-response alignment. When responsiveness declines, maintaining alignment requires a different signaling profile. In this context, increased signaling is not a sign of excess but an adjustment to altered interpretive conditions. The system shifts its output to preserve coordination, even as the underlying efficiency of signal translation has changed.

The Compensation Mechanism therefore alters how signaling patterns should be understood. Increased insulin signaling is not inherently indicative of increased regulatory strength, but instead reflects an attempt to offset reduced interpretive effectiveness. The signal does not become more powerful in its intrinsic capacity. It becomes more prominent in its presence to compensate for diminished responsiveness. This distinction separates compensation from amplification as an independent phenomenon, placing it within the adaptive structure of system behavior.

Compensation is not imposed from a central control point. It emerges through feedback interactions between signaling output and tissue-level response. As responses become less aligned with signaling input, feedback mechanisms adjust the level and persistence of signaling in an attempt to restore alignment. This creates a loop in which reduced responsiveness leads to increased signaling, which in turn modifies how tissues interpret subsequent signals. The loop is dynamic, continuously adjusting based on the evolving relationship between signal and response.

These feedback escalation loops define the structure of compensation over time. The system does not increase signaling once and return to baseline. It adjusts repeatedly, responding to the ongoing state of responsiveness. When increased signaling partially restores alignment, the system may stabilize at a new equilibrium with elevated output. When alignment remains incomplete, further adjustments occur, extending the escalation. This process reflects the system's attempt to maintain coherence within altered conditions rather than a movement toward a fixed endpoint.

The escalation loop introduces complexity into timing and interpretation. As signaling output increases, the temporal profile of signals changes. Signals may persist longer, overlap more frequently, or occur with altered spacing relative to prior patterns. These changes affect how signals are integrated into sequences, influencing how tissues interpret their meaning. Increased duration may blur the boundaries between signaling states, while increased frequency may alter the structure of temporal patterns. The result is a signaling environment that differs not only in magnitude but in temporal organization.

Coordination across tissues is reshaped under compensatory conditions. As signaling increases, tissues with reduced sensitivity may begin to respond more effectively, partially restoring their contribution to system behavior. At the same time, tissues with preserved or less altered sensitivity may respond more strongly to the increased signal, introducing asymmetry into coordination. This differential responsiveness alters the balance of contributions across tissues, affecting how energy is routed and how regulation is maintained. Coordination is preserved, but it is achieved through a different distribution of responses.

Partitioning reflects these changes in coordination. Increased signaling influences how energy is allocated across pathways, as tissues interpret the augmented signal within their respective contexts. In some domains, this may restore allocation patterns that had become attenuated under reduced sensitivity. In others, it may introduce shifts that reflect the altered balance of responsiveness across tissues. The resulting partitioning pattern is not identical to that observed under higher sensitivity. It is a new configuration that maintains functional outcomes through adjusted signaling and interpretation.

The Compensation Mechanism reveals that apparent stability can be maintained under conditions of underlying distortion. When increased signaling succeeds in restoring alignment between signal and response, observable outcomes may appear unchanged. Glucose regulation, energy distribution, and coordination across tissues may remain within functional ranges, suggesting stability. However, this stability is achieved through altered signaling dynamics, with increased output compensating for reduced responsiveness. The underlying system has changed, even if the observable behavior remains similar.

This distinction introduces the concept of hidden instability. Compensation can maintain outward alignment while internal dynamics shift toward greater complexity and strain. The system operates with increased signaling, altered timing, and modified coordination, all of which reflect a departure from the original interpretive framework. These changes may not produce immediate observable effects, but they alter the structure within which regulation occurs. Stability is preserved, but it is maintained through mechanisms that introduce additional demands on the system.

Hidden instability becomes more apparent over time as compensatory patterns persist. Repeated exposure to elevated signaling reinforces the adaptive adjustments that support compensation. Tissues adjust their responsiveness within this new context, potentially leading to further changes in sensitivity and interpretation. The system evolves within a framework of sustained compensation, with each adjustment influencing subsequent behavior. This evolution does not necessarily restore the original state. It establishes a new operating condition characterized by altered signaling and response dynamics.

The progression of compensation reflects the cumulative nature of these adaptations. As signaling patterns continue to adjust, the system may reach points at which further increases in output produce diminishing returns in restoring alignment. At this stage, the effectiveness of compensation begins to decline, even as signaling remains elevated. The feedback loop continues to operate, but its capacity to maintain stability becomes constrained by the limits of responsiveness within the system. The balance between signal and response becomes increasingly difficult to sustain.

Failure patterns within the Compensation Mechanism emerge when the system can no longer maintain alignment through increased signaling. This breakdown does not occur suddenly. It develops as the capacity for compensation is exceeded, leading to more pronounced divergence between signal and response. At this point, observable instability becomes more evident, as regulation can no longer be maintained within functional ranges through compensatory adjustments alone. The system transitions from masked instability to overt dysregulation.

The nature of this breakdown reflects the accumulated changes within the system. Prolonged signaling, altered timing, and modified coordination contribute to a state in which feedback loops operate under increased strain. Responses may become more variable, timing may become less precise, and partitioning may become less aligned with system demands. These changes represent the limits of compensation, demonstrating that adaptive mechanisms designed to preserve stability can, over time, contribute to its disruption when underlying conditions remain altered.

The Compensation Mechanism therefore defines compensation as both an adaptive response and a source of potential instability. It allows the system to maintain functional alignment under conditions of reduced sensitivity, extending stability through increased signaling. At the same time, it alters the structure of signaling dynamics, introducing changes that may accumulate and affect long-term behavior. Compensation does not resolve the underlying distortion. It manages its effects within the signaling framework.

The reframing inherent in this mechanism clarifies that increased signaling is not a direct indicator of increased regulatory capacity, but rather a reflection of the system's attempt to preserve alignment under reduced responsiveness. This reinterpretation shifts the focus from the magnitude of signaling to the relationship between signal and response, emphasizing that effectiveness is determined by translation rather than by output alone. Compensation emerges as a process that sustains function by adjusting this relationship, even as the underlying conditions that necessitate adjustment persist.

Within this framework, insulin continues to operate as a coordination signal, participating in the regulation of energy distribution and system behavior. The Compensation Mechanism defines how this participation changes when responsiveness declines, illustrating how the system adapts to maintain stability through altered signaling dynamics. It captures the interplay between adaptation and strain, demonstrating that the processes that preserve function in the short term can influence the trajectory of system behavior over longer periods.

The Spike vs Exposure Mechanism

The Spike vs Exposure Mechanism defines how insulin signaling must be understood as a pattern distributed across time rather than as a series of isolated events. It establishes that the metabolic system does not interpret individual signaling moments independently. It interprets cumulative exposure created by the interaction of signal magnitude, duration, frequency, and sequence. The distinction between a spike and exposure is not simply a difference in scale. It is a difference in how information is structured, integrated, and translated into system behavior.

A spike represents an acute signaling event, defined by a rapid increase in signal magnitude followed by a decline governed by clearance. It is a discrete occurrence with a definable beginning, peak, and resolution. Exposure represents the total signaling environment experienced over time, encompassing not only individual spikes but also their spacing, overlap, persistence, and repetition. While spikes are observable as individual events, exposure is the integrated effect of these events as they accumulate and interact within the system.

The system does not respond to spikes in isolation because interpretation is not reset between events. Each spike occurs within a context shaped by prior signals, residual activity, and ongoing coordination across tissues. This context defines how the spike is understood. A signal of identical magnitude may produce different responses depending on whether it follows a period of low exposure or occurs within an environment of sustained signaling. The spike itself does not carry sufficient information to determine its effect independently. Its meaning is derived from its position within cumulative exposure.

This relationship between spike and exposure alters how signaling should be interpreted. Insulin spikes are not the primary drivers of metabolic behavior, but instead are components of a broader exposure pattern that defines system response. This reframing shifts attention from the characteristics of individual events to the structure of signaling over time. It establishes that understanding metabolic behavior requires analysis of patterns rather than isolated measurements.

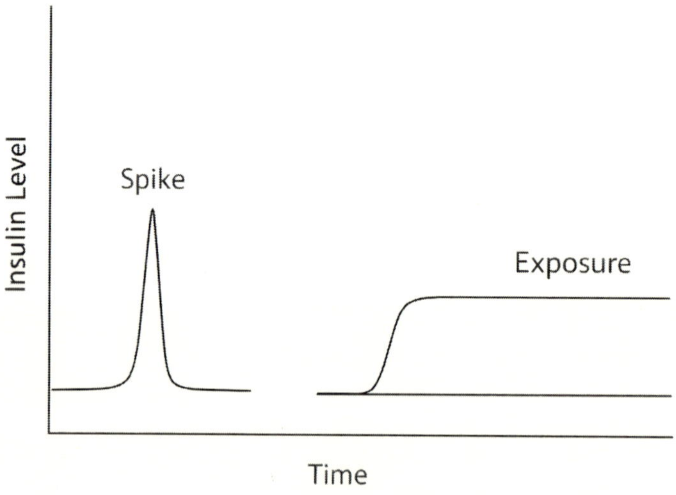

[Figure 5: Spike vs Exposure Comparison]

The distinction becomes more evident when considering that exposure incorporates multiple dimensions simultaneously. Magnitude contributes to exposure, but so does duration, determined by clearance. Frequency influences how often signals occur, while sequence determines how they are arranged relative to one another. These elements combine to create a signaling landscape that cannot be reduced to individual spikes. Exposure represents the integrated effect of this landscape, shaping how tissues interpret and respond to signals.

Timing plays a central role in the formation of exposure. The placement of spikes within time determines whether they are experienced as discrete events or as components of a sustained pattern. Closely spaced spikes may overlap due to incomplete clearance, creating extended periods of elevated signaling. Widely spaced spikes allow for clearer resolution between events, producing distinct signaling intervals. These differences alter the temporal structure of exposure, influencing how the system processes information.

Clearance defines the duration of each spike and therefore its contribution to exposure. A signal that resolves quickly contributes less to cumulative exposure than a signal that persists. When clearance is delayed, spikes extend in duration, increasing their overlap with subsequent signals and amplifying overall exposure. The system does not differentiate between exposure created by a single prolonged signal and exposure created by multiple overlapping signals. Both contribute to the same cumulative effect, shaping interpretation in similar ways.

Sequence integrates timing and clearance into a coherent pattern. The order in which spikes occur, and the intervals between them, determine how exposure evolves over time. Sequences can create patterns of sustained signaling, intermittent signaling, or irregular exposure, each of which produces different interpretive conditions. These conditions influence how tissues coordinate their responses, demonstrating that exposure is structured through the interaction of multiple temporal variables.

Repeated exposure influences sensitivity by shaping how tissues adjust their responsiveness to signaling patterns. When exposure is sustained or frequently repeated, tissues may adapt by modifying how they interpret signals, altering responsiveness to maintain stability under those conditions. These adaptations do not occur in response to individual spikes. They occur in response to the cumulative pattern of exposure, reflecting the system's integration of signaling over time.

Resistance emerges within this framework as a consequence of exposure patterns rather than as a response to isolated events. Sustained or repeated exposure alters interpretive frameworks, leading to progressive changes in responsiveness. These changes reflect adaptation to the signaling environment, demonstrating that resistance is linked to how signals are distributed across time rather than to their individual magnitude. The system responds to the pattern it experiences, adjusting sensitivity in relation to exposure rather than to spikes.

Compensation further illustrates the importance of exposure. As responsiveness declines under certain exposure patterns, signaling output increases to maintain alignment between signal and response. This increase contributes to overall exposure, reinforcing the pattern that led to adaptation. The feedback loop between exposure, responsiveness, and signaling output demonstrates that system behavior is shaped by cumulative effects rather than by isolated events. Each component influences the others, creating a dynamic interaction that evolves over time.

Focusing on individual spikes obscures this interaction. When analysis is limited to discrete events, the broader pattern of exposure is not captured. This can lead to interpretations that attribute system behavior to specific spikes without considering the cumulative context in which those spikes occur. Such interpretations fail to account for the temporal structure of signaling, leading to incomplete or inaccurate understanding of metabolic dynamics.

The system integrates exposure into coordination across tissues. Muscle, liver, and adipose tissue do not respond to spikes independently. They respond to the exposure pattern created by the sequence of signals they experience. This pattern shapes how each tissue interprets current signals, influencing how they contribute to energy routing, partitioning, and regulation. Coordination emerges from the alignment of these responses within the shared exposure environment.

Partitioning is directly influenced by exposure patterns. Sustained exposure may promote allocation strategies that differ from those observed under intermittent exposure, as tissues interpret prolonged signaling as indicative of continuous availability. Intermittent exposure may produce distinct allocation patterns, reflecting the alternation between signaling states. These differences demonstrate that partitioning outcomes are determined by the structure of exposure rather than by the characteristics of individual spikes.

Feedback regulation operates within the context of exposure as well. The feedback loop between glucose and insulin is influenced by the cumulative pattern of signaling, with exposure shaping how signals are generated and how responses are integrated. Sustained exposure may alter the dynamics of feedback, extending the period over which signals influence regulation. Intermittent exposure may produce more discrete feedback cycles, affecting how the system maintains stability across time. These variations reflect the influence of exposure on regulatory processes.

Failure patterns within the Spike vs Exposure Mechanism arise when cumulative exposure is misinterpreted or ignored. When emphasis is placed on individual spikes, the broader pattern of signaling may remain unrecognized, leading to incomplete understanding of system behavior. This can result in misalignment between interpretation and actual conditions, as the system's responses are shaped by exposure rather than by isolated events.

Misinterpretation of exposure can lead to underestimation of cumulative effects. When individual spikes appear within expected ranges, the overall exposure pattern may still produce conditions that influence sensitivity, resistance, and compensation. Without accounting for cumulative exposure, these effects may not be attributed to their underlying cause. The system's behavior may appear inconsistent when viewed through the lens of isolated events, as the cumulative pattern that defines interpretation is not considered.

Distortion also arises when exposure patterns become irregular or misaligned. Inconsistent timing, delayed clearance, or overlapping signals can create exposure environments that challenge the system's ability to establish stable interpretive frameworks. These conditions introduce variability into coordination, partitioning, and regulation, as tissues adjust to changing patterns without a consistent structure. The resulting behavior reflects the system's attempt to manage exposure variability rather than the effect of individual spikes.

The Spike vs Exposure Mechanism therefore establishes that metabolic behavior is determined by the pattern of signaling over time. Insulin spikes are components of this pattern, but they do not define it independently. Exposure integrates magnitude, duration, frequency, and sequence into a unified framework that shapes interpretation and response. Understanding this mechanism requires shifting focus from discrete events to the structure of signaling across time.

Within this framework, stability is maintained when exposure patterns align with system conditions, allowing tissues to interpret signals consistently and coordinate their responses effectively. Instability arises when exposure patterns are misaligned, irregular, or misunderstood, leading to variability in interpretation and response. The mechanism captures the dynamic relationship between spikes and exposure, demonstrating that long-term behavior emerges from cumulative patterns rather than from isolated events.

The Baseline Elevation Mechanism

The Baseline Elevation Mechanism defines how the metabolic system transitions from interpreting insulin signaling as a sequence of discrete events to operating within a persistently elevated signaling environment that reshapes the meaning of all subsequent inputs. It describes the gradual upward drift of baseline signaling levels and the resulting shift in how signals are integrated, separated, and translated into coordinated behavior. This mechanism does not depend on the magnitude of individual spikes. It depends on the cumulative pattern of exposure that prevents full return to baseline, establishing a new reference state from which all signaling is interpreted.

Acute fluctuations in insulin signaling are characterized by identifiable rises and declines that allow the system to distinguish between periods of active signaling and relative absence. These fluctuations create temporal contrast, enabling tissues to interpret signals as part of a sequence with defined boundaries. Baseline elevation alters this structure by reducing the distinction between these periods. When the signal does not fully resolve, the system remains in a state of partial activation, and subsequent signals are layered onto an already elevated baseline rather than emerging from a lower reference point.

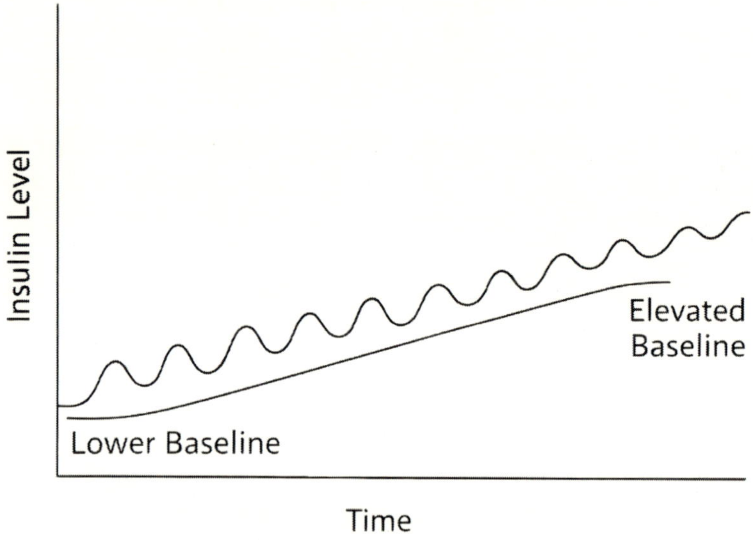

[Figure 6: Baseline Elevation Over Time]

This shift introduces a new condition in which baseline signaling level becomes the primary determinant of system state. System state is not defined by spikes, but by baseline signaling level. This reframing changes how signaling patterns are interpreted. Individual spikes no longer represent transitions between distinct states. They become variations within a continuous field of activation, with their relative impact diminished by the elevated baseline from which they arise.

The drift in baseline signaling occurs through repeated exposure patterns that prevent complete clearance between signals. When signals occur with sufficient frequency or duration, residual activity persists, and the system does not return to its prior baseline before the next signal arrives. Over time, this accumulation raises the baseline level, creating a sustained environment of signaling that differs from the intermittent structure observed under conditions of full resolution. The process is gradual, reflecting the cumulative effect of overlapping signals and incomplete recovery between them.

This elevated baseline alters the interpretive environment across all tissues. Muscle, liver, and adipose tissue do not interpret signals in isolation. They interpret them relative to the current baseline. When baseline signaling is elevated, the threshold for distinguishing new signals changes. A signal that would represent a significant increase from a lower baseline may represent only a marginal change from an elevated one. The informational contrast between signals is reduced, altering how tissues translate signaling into coordinated action.

Timing is directly affected by this shift. The separation between signals becomes less distinct as baseline elevation increases. Signals overlap not only due to their immediate duration but also because they are superimposed on a background of persistent activation. This reduces the clarity of temporal sequences, making it more difficult for the system to differentiate between discrete events. The temporal structure that once defined signaling patterns becomes compressed, with intervals between signals losing their interpretive significance.

Clearance plays a central role in this process by determining how fully signals resolve. When clearance is efficient, signals return toward baseline, preserving temporal distinction. When clearance is incomplete or delayed, residual signaling contributes to baseline elevation, extending the period of activation beyond the initial event. As this pattern repeats, the system shifts toward a state in which signals no longer define clear boundaries but instead contribute to a continuous signaling environment.

The persistence of this environment creates a continuous activation state across tissues. Muscle tissue operates under conditions in which signaling influence remains present, altering how it interprets subsequent inputs and how it allocates energy toward use. The liver adjusts its regulation of circulating substrates within this sustained signaling context, influencing how availability is maintained. Adipose tissue interprets the persistent signal as an ongoing condition rather than as a discrete event, modifying its buffering behavior accordingly. These changes occur simultaneously, reshaping coordination across the system.

Sensitivity is influenced by this continuous activation state. When signaling remains elevated, tissues may adjust their responsiveness to manage the sustained input. This adjustment reflects adaptation to the new baseline, altering how signals are translated into action. Sensitivity does not decline in response to individual spikes. It adjusts in response to the persistent signaling environment created by baseline elevation. The result is a change in how tissues interpret both baseline and incremental signals.

Resistance emerges within this framework as a consequence of altered interpretive conditions. When baseline signaling is elevated, the system may adjust its responsiveness to maintain stability within this environment. This adjustment reduces the clarity of signal-response alignment, contributing to the progressive distortion described in the Resistance Mechanism. The elevated baseline therefore acts as a driver of changes in responsiveness, linking exposure patterns to the evolution of resistance.

Compensation interacts with baseline elevation by increasing signaling output in response to reduced responsiveness. As sensitivity declines, signaling output rises to maintain alignment between signal and response. This increased output contributes to further elevation of the baseline, reinforcing the persistent activation state. The interaction between compensation and baseline elevation creates a feedback dynamic in which increased signaling both responds to and amplifies the conditions that necessitate it.

Exposure is redefined under conditions of baseline elevation. Rather than being composed of discrete spikes separated by periods of lower activity, exposure becomes continuous, with incremental variations occurring within an already elevated field. The distinction between spike and exposure diminishes, as spikes no longer represent isolated contributions to cumulative signaling. Instead, they become fluctuations within a sustained exposure pattern that defines the system's interpretive context.

Partitioning is reshaped by this continuous exposure. Allocation of energy across use, circulation, and storage is influenced by the persistent signaling environment, as tissues interpret sustained availability differently than intermittent availability. The balance between pathways shifts in response to the altered interpretive framework, producing allocation patterns that reflect the continuous activation state. These patterns are not determined by individual signals but by the baseline condition within which those signals are interpreted.

Feedback regulation is also affected by baseline elevation. The interaction between glucose and insulin signaling operates within a loop that depends on the clarity of signal-response relationships. When baseline signaling is elevated, the distinction between changes in glucose and corresponding signaling adjustments becomes less pronounced. Feedback loops may operate over extended durations, with signals persisting beyond the conditions that initiated them. This alters the timing and magnitude of feedback responses, influencing how effectively the system maintains stability.

Coordination across tissues is modified as each component adapts to the elevated baseline. Muscle, liver, and adipose tissue align their responses within a shared environment of persistent signaling, but their contributions may shift as responsiveness changes. The balance of allocation and regulation reflects these adjustments, producing coordinated behavior that differs from that observed under conditions of lower baseline signaling. The system remains coordinated, but the nature of coordination evolves with the baseline.

Failure patterns associated with baseline elevation arise from the loss of signal distinction and the persistence of activation. When signals cannot be clearly separated, interpretation becomes less precise, and coordination becomes more complex. The system may rely increasingly on compensatory mechanisms to maintain alignment, introducing additional strain into the signaling framework. As baseline elevation continues, the capacity for discrete regulation diminishes, and variability may increase as the system operates within a compressed range of interpretive states.

Chronic elevation can lead to a condition in which individual spikes become less meaningful within overall exposure. Their contribution to the signaling environment is small relative to the elevated baseline, reducing their ability to convey distinct information. This diminishes the system's capacity to use spikes as indicators of change, as the background level of signaling dominates interpretation. The system becomes less responsive to incremental variation, relying instead on broader patterns of exposure to guide behavior.

The Baseline Elevation Mechanism therefore defines how sustained changes in signaling environment reshape the structure of metabolic regulation. It establishes that baseline signaling level determines the context within which all signals are interpreted, influencing timing, clearance, sensitivity, resistance, compensation, and coordination. By shifting the system from discrete signaling states to continuous activation, it alters the way information is processed and how responses are organized across tissues.

Within this framework, insulin remains a coordination signal that communicates energy availability. Its role is not diminished by baseline elevation, but its interpretation is transformed. The system operates within a different reference state, and the meaning of signals is derived from their relationship to this state rather than from their isolated characteristics. Stability and instability emerge from how the system adapts to this persistent environment, demonstrating that baseline signaling level is a defining feature of metabolic behavior over time.

The Variability Mechanism

The Variability Mechanism defines how the structure of insulin signaling fluctuates across time and how those fluctuations influence the system's ability to maintain coordinated, interpretable behavior. It establishes that change within the metabolic system is not inherently destabilizing. The system depends on fluctuation to regulate energy distribution, adjust to shifting conditions, and maintain dynamic stability. Variability becomes significant when fluctuation loses its structured form, altering the clarity and predictability of signaling patterns.

Fluctuation is an expected characteristic of a signaling system that operates continuously. Insulin levels rise and fall in response to changes in energy availability, and these changes create oscillatory patterns that tissues interpret as part of coordinated regulation. These oscillations are not random. They follow temporal structures defined by timing, sequence, and clearance, allowing the system to distinguish between different signaling states. Controlled fluctuation maintains this structure, preserving the interpretive clarity required for coordination across tissues.

Variability emerges when these oscillatory patterns become irregular, inconsistent, or fragmented. The distinction between fluctuation and variability is not based on the presence of change but on the organization of that change. Variability is not the presence of change, but the loss of structured change. This reframing shifts attention from whether signals fluctuate to how those fluctuations are organized across time. Structured oscillations support stability, while disorganized variability reduces the system's ability to interpret signals consistently.

Oscillation patterns represent structured fluctuation, where signals rise and fall within predictable ranges and sequences. These patterns allow tissues to anticipate and align their responses, maintaining coordination through repeated cycles of signaling and resolution. The system integrates these cycles into a coherent framework, enabling efficient translation of signals into action. Stability within this framework is dynamic, reflecting the system's capacity to manage continuous change through organized patterns.

Destabilizing variability differs from oscillation in that it disrupts this organization. Signals may vary in magnitude, duration, and timing without consistent relationships between them. Intervals between signals may become irregular, clearance may vary unpredictably, and sequences may lose continuity. These changes alter the temporal structure of signaling, making it more difficult for tissues to interpret signals within a stable framework. The system continues to fluctuate, but the fluctuations no longer carry consistent meaning.

Variability is not random error. It is a structural property of the signaling system that reflects how signals are generated, distributed, and resolved. Changes in sensitivity, resistance, compensation, exposure, and baseline elevation all contribute to the emergence of variability by altering how signals are produced and interpreted. The resulting patterns reflect the interaction of these mechanisms rather than isolated disturbances. Variability therefore provides information about the state of the system, indicating how well signaling patterns maintain coherence under changing conditions.

The effect of variability on interpretation is central to the mechanism. Tissues rely on consistent patterns to translate signals into coordinated responses. When patterns become irregular, the relationship between signal and meaning becomes less clear. A signal of a given magnitude may be interpreted differently depending on its temporal context, and when that context is unstable, interpretation becomes less reliable. This introduces variability into tissue-level responses, as each tissue attempts to interpret signals within a shifting framework.

Excessive variability reduces signal clarity by diminishing the distinction between different signaling states. When signals vary unpredictably, the system cannot establish stable thresholds for interpretation. The contrast between rising and falling phases may become less defined, and the boundaries between signals may become blurred. This reduces the system's ability to distinguish between conditions, affecting how signals are translated into action. Clarity depends on consistent relationships between signals, and variability disrupts those relationships.

Timing is directly affected by variability through the disruption of temporal sequences. In a structured system, signals occur in patterns that allow for predictable integration across time. Variability alters these patterns, introducing irregular intervals and inconsistent sequencing. This affects how signals overlap and how they are spaced, complicating the system's ability to construct coherent sequences. As timing becomes less predictable, coordination across tissues becomes more difficult, as responses no longer align within a shared temporal framework.

Coordination depends on the alignment of tissue-level responses to shared signaling patterns. When variability increases, tissues may interpret signals differently based on their local context and recent exposure. This divergence introduces inconsistency into coordination, as responses may occur at different times or with different intensities across tissues. The resulting behavior reflects a system in which alignment is reduced, requiring additional adjustments to maintain functional stability.

Partitioning is influenced by variability through its effect on allocation decisions. When signaling patterns are consistent, allocation across use, circulation, and storage follows predictable structures. Variability disrupts these structures, introducing fluctuations in how energy is distributed across pathways. These fluctuations may not align with current system conditions, producing imbalances that affect both immediate function and long-term stability. The system continues to allocate energy, but the distribution becomes less coherent.

Sensitivity interacts with variability by shaping how tissues respond to irregular patterns. Changes in responsiveness may amplify or dampen the effects of variability, depending on how tissues adjust to the signaling environment. When sensitivity varies across tissues, the impact of variability on coordination is further increased, as each tissue interprets signals within its own responsive context. Resistance contributes to this process by altering the fidelity of signal interpretation, increasing the likelihood that variability will produce divergent responses.

Compensation influences variability through its effect on signaling output. As the system increases signaling to maintain alignment under reduced sensitivity, the structure of signaling patterns may change. Increased output can alter timing, duration, and sequence, contributing to variability in how signals are experienced across tissues. These changes interact with baseline elevation, where sustained signaling reduces the distinction between signals and increases the likelihood of irregular overlap. The combined effect of these mechanisms shapes the variability observed within the system.

Exposure patterns are closely linked to variability, as they define the cumulative structure of signaling across time. When exposure is consistent, variability is constrained within predictable bounds, allowing the system to maintain coherence. When exposure becomes irregular, variability increases, reflecting the lack of stable patterns. The system adapts to these conditions, but the adaptation may introduce further changes in responsiveness and coordination, reinforcing variability over time.

Feedback regulation is affected by variability through its influence on the coupling between signals and responses. The feedback loop relies on predictable relationships between changes in glucose and corresponding adjustments in insulin signaling. Variability disrupts these relationships, introducing delays, inconsistencies, or exaggerated responses. This alters the structure of feedback cycles, affecting how effectively the system can maintain stability. As predictability decreases, the system must rely on broader adjustments rather than precise regulation.

Predictability is a key outcome of structured signaling. When variability increases, predictability decreases, and the system's ability to anticipate and align responses is reduced. This does not mean that the system becomes entirely unpredictable. It means that the range of possible responses expands, and the relationship between signals and outcomes becomes less consistent. The system continues to function, but with increased variability in how it responds to similar conditions.

Failure patterns within the Variability Mechanism arise when variability exceeds the system's capacity to maintain coherence. At this stage, the loss of structured change leads to significant disruption in timing, coordination, and partitioning. Signals may no longer produce consistent responses, and feedback regulation may become increasingly unstable. The system may rely more heavily on compensatory mechanisms, further altering signaling patterns and contributing to additional variability.

These failure patterns reflect the cumulative effect of disrupted signaling structure. Variability is not the cause of instability in isolation. It is the expression of underlying changes in how signals are generated, interpreted, and coordinated. As these changes accumulate, the system moves further from structured oscillation toward irregular fluctuation, reducing its ability to maintain stability through organized patterns.

The Variability Mechanism therefore defines how the organization of signaling fluctuations determines the system's capacity for stable behavior. It emphasizes that change is not inherently destabilizing, but that the structure of change is critical. By distinguishing between controlled oscillation and disorganized variability, the mechanism provides a framework for understanding how signaling patterns influence interpretation, coordination, and regulation across tissues.

Within this framework, insulin remains a coordination signal that operates within a dynamic environment of continuous fluctuation. The effectiveness of this signaling depends on the preservation of structured patterns that allow for consistent interpretation. As variability increases and structure is lost, the system's ability to translate signals into coordinated action is diminished, demonstrating that stability depends on the integrity of signaling organization over time.

The Nutrition Interaction Mechanism

The Nutrition Interaction Mechanism defines how food functions as an input to the metabolic system that influences signaling behavior without independently determining outcomes. It establishes that nutrition does not operate as a direct driver of metabolic results. Instead, it interacts with the signaling layer by shaping the structure, timing, magnitude, and sequence of insulin signaling. These signals are then interpreted within the context of the system's current state, producing outcomes that reflect interaction rather than direct causation.

Food enters the system as a variable input that alters the conditions under which signaling occurs. This input does not act in isolation. It modifies the signaling environment by influencing how insulin is generated, how long it persists, and how it is distributed across time. The effect of this input depends on how it is integrated into the existing signaling framework, which is already shaped by prior exposure, baseline conditions, sensitivity, and coordination across tissues. The Nutrition Interaction Mechanism therefore situates food within the broader system as a contributor to signaling patterns rather than as an independent determinant of metabolic behavior.

The distinction between input patterns and isolated intake events is central to this mechanism. A single instance of intake can produce a measurable signaling response, but this response is interpreted within the context of preceding and subsequent inputs. Input patterns describe how food is distributed across time, including frequency, spacing, and composition. These patterns create structured exposure environments that shape how signals are generated and how they accumulate. The system does not respond to isolated events independently. It responds to the pattern created by those events as they interact across time.

This distinction leads to a reframing of how food should be understood within the system. Food does not directly determine metabolic outcomes; it shapes signaling patterns that are interpreted by the system. This interpretation depends on the existing conditions within the system, including baseline signaling level, responsiveness, and prior exposure. The same input can therefore produce different signaling responses depending on when it occurs, how it is sequenced, and the state of the system at the time of input.

Input patterns influence the structure of insulin signaling across multiple dimensions. Timing determines when signals are initiated relative to existing patterns. Magnitude reflects the amplitude of the signaling response to a given input. Duration is shaped by clearance, determining how long the signal persists. Sequence defines how signals are arranged relative to one another, influencing overlap and separation. These dimensions combine to create a signaling profile that reflects the interaction between input and system state.

The influence of input on signaling is not uniform across conditions. A given input may produce a distinct signaling response in a system with low baseline signaling compared to one with elevated baseline conditions. When baseline is low, signals may emerge as discrete events with clear boundaries, allowing for structured oscillation. When baseline is elevated, the same input may produce a signal that is layered onto an existing field of activation, reducing contrast and altering interpretation. The input itself does not change. The system's response to that input changes based on its current state.

Sensitivity further modifies how inputs influence signaling. In a system with higher responsiveness, a given input may produce a signal that is translated efficiently into coordinated action, with minimal distortion. In a system with reduced responsiveness, the same input may produce a signal that requires amplification through compensation, altering its magnitude and duration. These changes affect how the signal contributes to exposure, demonstrating that input interacts with sensitivity to shape signaling patterns.

Resistance emerges within this interaction as a consequence of how repeated input patterns influence responsiveness over time. Sustained or frequent inputs can contribute to exposure patterns that alter sensitivity, leading to changes in how signals are interpreted. These changes do not occur in response to individual inputs. They develop through cumulative interaction between input patterns and system adaptation. The resulting resistance reflects the system's adjustment to the signaling environment created by those patterns.

Compensation further integrates into this framework by adjusting signaling output in response to altered responsiveness. As sensitivity declines, the system may increase signaling in response to input to maintain alignment between signal and response. This increased signaling contributes to exposure and baseline elevation, reinforcing the interaction between input patterns and system state. The effect of input is therefore mediated through multiple layers of interaction, each influencing how signals are generated and interpreted.

Baseline elevation represents a condition in which input patterns contribute to sustained signaling environments. When inputs occur with sufficient frequency or duration, signals may not fully resolve, leading to persistent elevation. In this state, new inputs interact with an already elevated baseline, altering how signals are generated and interpreted. The distinction between discrete responses and continuous exposure becomes less pronounced, and input contributes to maintaining a persistent activation state rather than producing isolated events.

Variability is also influenced by input patterns. When inputs are structured and consistent, they contribute to stable signaling patterns that support predictable interpretation. When inputs are irregular, they introduce variability into signaling, affecting timing, sequence, and magnitude. This variability interacts with other mechanisms, influencing coordination and partitioning across tissues. The resulting signaling patterns reflect the combined effect of input variability and system responsiveness.

Partitioning is shaped by how input-driven signals are interpreted within the system. Inputs influence the availability of energy, but the allocation of that energy across use, circulation, and storage depends on how signals are processed. When signals are interpreted within a stable framework, partitioning aligns with system demands. When interpretation is altered by factors such as baseline elevation or variability, partitioning may shift, producing allocation patterns that differ from those expected under more stable conditions.

Feedback regulation integrates input with signaling through the interaction between glucose and insulin dynamics. Inputs influence circulating glucose levels, which in turn affect insulin signaling. This interaction forms part of the feedback loop that regulates energy availability. The structure of this loop is influenced by input patterns, as timing, magnitude, and duration of inputs shape how signals are generated and how responses are integrated. The system does not respond to input independently of this loop. It responds to how input interacts with feedback processes.

The Nutrition Interaction Mechanism therefore establishes that inputs shape signaling behavior over time through their influence on patterns rather than through isolated effects. This shaping occurs without prescribing specific actions or outcomes. It reflects the system's integration of input with existing conditions, producing signaling patterns that are interpreted within a dynamic framework. The effect of input is always conditional, depending on how it interacts with the system's current state and history of exposure.

Failure patterns arise when inputs are interpreted without reference to system context. When food is treated as an independent driver of outcomes, the interaction between input and signaling is overlooked. This can lead to assumptions that identical inputs will produce identical outcomes, ignoring the role of baseline conditions, sensitivity, and exposure patterns. Such interpretations fail to account for the variability observed in system behavior, as they do not consider the dynamic nature of signaling interaction.

Misinterpretation also occurs when input patterns are reduced to isolated events rather than understood as part of a sequence. This approach overlooks how repeated inputs shape exposure and influence adaptation over time. Without considering patterns, the system's response may appear inconsistent or unpredictable, as the cumulative context that defines interpretation is not recognized. The result is an incomplete understanding of how input interacts with signaling to produce outcomes.

The Nutrition Interaction Mechanism therefore bridges the signaling model with real-world inputs by situating food within the system as a modulator of signaling patterns. It clarifies that inputs do not act independently but interact with a complex network of mechanisms that determine how signals are generated, interpreted, and translated into coordinated behavior. By maintaining a signal-based framing, it preserves analytical neutrality while providing a structured understanding of how input contributes to metabolic dynamics.

Within this framework, food remains an input that influences the system without dictating its outcomes. Its effect is mediated through signaling patterns that are shaped by timing, sequence, and interaction with system state. Stability and instability emerge from how these patterns are interpreted and integrated, demonstrating that the role of nutrition is defined not by its direct effects but by its interaction with the signaling architecture of the metabolic system.

The Fasting Interaction Mechanism

The Fasting Interaction Mechanism defines how periods of reduced or low insulin signaling function as integral components of metabolic regulation, shaping the interpretive environment through the structured absence of signal. It establishes that the system does not operate solely through the presence of signaling but through the alternation between signaling states, where both presence and absence contribute to coordination. These periods of reduced signaling are not interruptions to system function. They are conditions within which the system recalibrates, resolves prior signals, and restores the capacity for clear interpretation.

Fasting is not an intervention; it is a signaling condition in which absence of insulin becomes part of regulation. This reframing removes the concept of fasting from a behavioral or prescriptive framework and situates it within the signaling architecture of the system. In this context, fasting is defined by the reduction of insulin signaling toward lower levels, creating a temporal environment in which the system operates under different interpretive conditions than those present during active signaling. The absence of signal is not empty. It carries informational significance by altering how subsequent signals are received and integrated.

Periods of reduced signaling occur as part of the natural oscillation of the system. When inputs are not introduced, insulin signaling declines through clearance processes, allowing the system to move toward lower baseline conditions. This decline is not instantaneous. It unfolds over time, reflecting the resolution of prior signals and the progressive reduction of their interpretive influence. As signaling diminishes, the system transitions into a state where the absence of signal becomes the dominant condition, shaping how tissues interpret their environment.

Signal suppression contributes to resetting interpretive conditions by restoring temporal distinction between signaling states. When signals fully resolve, tissues regain the ability to differentiate clearly between periods of presence and absence. This distinction supports structured oscillation, enabling the system to maintain coherence in timing and sequence. Without sufficient suppression, signals overlap and persist, reducing the clarity of interpretation. The reduction of signaling therefore plays a critical role in preserving the structural integrity of the signaling framework.

The effect of reduced signaling on baseline is central to this mechanism. As insulin levels decline, baseline signaling moves toward lower levels, re-establishing a reference point from which future signals can emerge. This reset does not return the system to a static state. It creates conditions under which new signals can be interpreted with greater contrast relative to baseline. When baseline is elevated, signals are layered onto a persistent field of activation. When baseline is reduced, signals emerge from a clearer background, enhancing their interpretive significance.

Exposure patterns are reshaped during periods of low signaling. Rather than continuous exposure defined by overlapping signals, the system experiences intervals of reduced activity that interrupt cumulative patterns. These intervals alter how exposure is integrated over time, creating segments within which signaling can be differentiated. The system does not interpret exposure as a continuous field under these conditions. It interprets it as a sequence with defined transitions, improving the coherence of signaling patterns.

Signal separation is enhanced when reduced signaling allows for distinct intervals between events. Clearance processes complete their function, and residual signaling diminishes, preventing overlap between successive signals. This separation preserves the temporal structure required for accurate interpretation. When separation is insufficient, signals blend into one another, reducing the system's ability to distinguish between conditions. The presence of low-signal intervals therefore supports the maintenance of structured timing within the system.

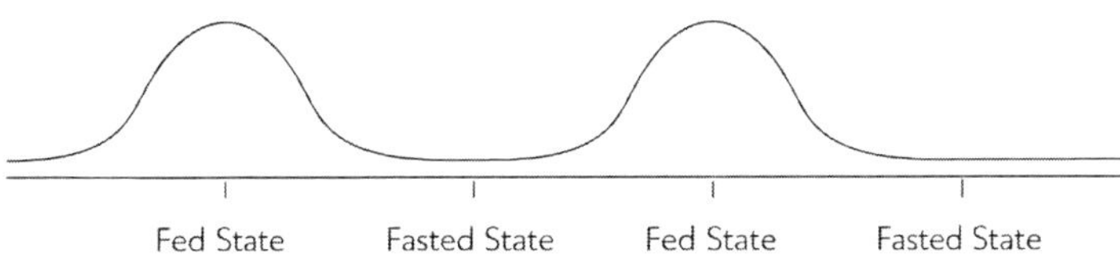

[Figure 7: Fed–Fasted Insulin Cycle]

Recovery dynamics emerge as signaling returns following periods of suppression. When new inputs are introduced, insulin signaling rises from a lower baseline, producing a signal that is interpreted within a restored context. This transition is not simply a reversal of suppression. It is a reintegration of signaling into a system that has undergone a period of reduced activity. The resulting signal is interpreted relative to the absence that preceded it, enhancing its informational clarity and influencing how tissues coordinate their responses.

Reintegration involves the alignment of signaling with the system's current state following suppression. Tissues do not respond to returning signals in the same way they respond to signals within sustained exposure conditions. The reduced baseline alters sensitivity, timing, and coordination, affecting how signals are translated into action. Reintegration therefore represents a transition between signaling states, where the system adjusts from absence to presence within a structured temporal sequence.

Sensitivity is influenced by periods of reduced signaling through the recalibration of responsiveness. When signaling remains low for sufficient intervals, tissues may adjust their interpretive frameworks, altering how they respond to subsequent signals. This adjustment reflects the system's adaptation to the absence of signal, restoring the capacity for efficient translation when signals reappear. The relationship between sensitivity and fasting is therefore mediated through the effect of reduced signaling on interpretive conditions rather than through direct alteration of the signal itself.

Resistance is also shaped by these dynamics. When signaling is persistently elevated, interpretive distortion may develop as described in prior mechanisms. Periods of reduced signaling alter this environment by interrupting sustained exposure, modifying how signals are integrated over time. These interruptions influence the progression of resistance by altering the patterns that drive adaptation. Resistance is not reversed or eliminated in a discrete manner. It is influenced by the structure of signaling patterns, including the presence of low-signal intervals.

Compensation interacts with fasting through its effect on signaling output. In conditions where compensation has elevated signaling to maintain alignment, periods of reduced input allow for the decline of this elevated output. This decline affects the feedback loops that drive compensation, altering the relationship between signal and response. The system may adjust its output in response to reduced signaling, reflecting the integration of fasting within the broader signaling framework. The interaction between compensation and reduced signaling demonstrates that absence influences not only baseline but also the dynamics of signaling output.

Variability is influenced by the presence or absence of structured low-signal intervals. When periods of reduced signaling are consistent and aligned with system conditions, they contribute to structured oscillation, supporting stability. When these periods are irregular or insufficient, variability increases, as signals overlap and temporal patterns lose coherence. The integration of low-signal intervals therefore plays a role in maintaining the structure of fluctuation within the system.

Coordination across tissues depends on the alignment of signaling patterns, including both presence and absence. When low-signal intervals are integrated consistently, tissues can align their responses within a shared temporal framework. Muscle, liver, and adipose tissue interpret the absence of signal as part of the sequence, adjusting their behavior accordingly. This alignment supports coordinated transitions between states of activity and recovery. When absence is misaligned or insufficient, coordination becomes more complex, as tissues operate within different interpretive contexts.

Partitioning is also affected by reduced signaling. During periods of low insulin signaling, allocation patterns shift as tissues interpret the absence of signal within their functional roles. These shifts reflect the system's adaptation to reduced availability, influencing how energy is distributed across pathways. When signaling returns, partitioning adjusts again, reflecting the reintegration of signals into the system. The alternation between these states contributes to the overall pattern of energy allocation across time.

Failure patterns within the Fasting Interaction Mechanism arise when periods of reduced signaling are insufficient, inconsistent, or misaligned with system conditions. When signals do not fully resolve, baseline remains elevated, and the system does not achieve the reset required for clear interpretation. This leads to persistent overlap between signals, reducing temporal distinction and contributing to variability. When low-signal intervals are irregular, the system cannot establish consistent oscillation patterns, affecting coordination and predictability.

Misalignment occurs when the timing of reduced signaling does not correspond with the system's broader regulatory structure. In such cases, the absence of signal may not integrate effectively into the sequence, reducing its ability to restore interpretive clarity. The system continues to function, but the benefits of structured absence are diminished, and signaling patterns may become less coherent over time.

The Fasting Interaction Mechanism therefore defines how the absence of insulin signaling contributes to metabolic regulation by shaping the temporal structure within which signals are interpreted. It establishes that both presence and absence are required for coherent signaling patterns, and that periods of reduced signaling play a critical role in maintaining the system's capacity for accurate interpretation and coordination.

Within this framework, fasting is understood as a condition that alters the signaling environment rather than as an action that produces outcomes directly. Its role is defined by how it interacts with the signaling architecture, influencing baseline, exposure, sensitivity, and coordination. The system's behavior reflects the integration of these interactions, demonstrating that absence is not a void within the system but a structured component of its regulatory process.

The Stress Interaction Mechanism

The Stress Interaction Mechanism defines how externally generated signals enter the metabolic system as modifiers of the signaling environment rather than as direct drivers of metabolic outcomes. Stress-related inputs do not determine energy allocation, glucose regulation, or signaling behavior independently. They alter the conditions within which insulin signaling is produced, interpreted, and coordinated. This establishes an interaction layer in which external signals influence internal processes by reshaping the context of signaling rather than by replacing or overriding it.

This interaction layer is continuous rather than episodic. External signals are integrated into the system alongside internal signals, forming a composite environment in which interpretation occurs. Under stable conditions, this integration preserves coherence, allowing insulin signaling to maintain its role as a coordination signal. Under distortion, external inputs alter the structure of this environment, introducing competing influences that modify how signals are weighted and translated into action. The mechanism therefore begins with the recognition that stress operates through modification of context, not through direct execution of metabolic effects.

The indirect modulation framework defines how these external signals influence system behavior. Stress does not act directly on metabolic pathways. It alters the interpretive environment by changing the relative weighting of signals, modifying the temporal structure of signaling, and influencing how tissues prioritize information. These changes are conditional, depending on baseline signaling levels, exposure patterns, and the current state of responsiveness across tissues. The same external input can therefore produce different outcomes depending on the system into which it is introduced.

Under normal conditions, this modulation remains within a range that preserves system coherence. External signals are integrated without disrupting the structure of signaling sequences, allowing the system to maintain coordinated responses. Under distortion, the modulation alters key structural features such as timing, sequence, and signal separation. The system continues to function, but the conditions under which signals are interpreted shift, introducing variability into coordination and response. The outcome reflects the interaction between external input and internal state rather than the direct effect of the input itself.

The interaction between cortisol and insulin illustrates how parallel signaling systems intersect within this framework. Cortisol modifies the context of glucose availability, influencing how insulin signaling is interpreted without directly opposing it. The two signals operate within the same interpretive environment, contributing different informational inputs that must be integrated. Under normal conditions, this integration allows for coordinated regulation, with each signal contributing to a balanced representation of system state.

When this interaction becomes distorted, the relative weighting of these signals changes. Cortisol-related signaling may alter how insulin signals are interpreted, shifting the emphasis placed on availability versus demand. This does not eliminate insulin's role but modifies its influence within the system. The effect on interpretation is a change in how signals are translated into coordinated responses, while the effect on coordination is a redistribution of response priorities across tissues. The system adapts to this altered weighting, but the resulting behavior reflects the modified interaction rather than the original signal structure.

Signaling layer interference emerges when multiple inputs compete within the interpretive environment. Each signal contributes information, but the system must determine how to prioritize and integrate these inputs. Under normal conditions, this integration produces coherent interpretation, with signals reinforcing or complementing one another. Under distortion, competition between signals alters their relative influence, creating ambiguity in interpretation and shifting the priorities that guide coordination.

This interference propagates into coordination by altering how tissues align their responses. When signal weighting becomes inconsistent, tissues may interpret the same signaling environment differently, leading to divergence in behavior. The resulting coordination impact is a reduction in alignment across tissues, while the interpretive effect is an increase in ambiguity regarding signal meaning. The system continues to operate, but coherence is reduced, requiring additional adjustments to maintain functional outcomes.

Sleep disruption introduces a breakdown in timing structure, affecting how signals are sequenced and resolved. The system depends on consistent temporal organization to maintain structured oscillation. When this organization is disrupted, signals occur with altered spacing and duration, affecting how they overlap and interact. Under normal conditions, timing supports clear separation between signals, preserving interpretive clarity. Under distortion, misalignment introduces overlap and irregularity, reducing the precision of temporal sequences.

These timing changes propagate into downstream coordination. Overlapping signals reduce the ability of tissues to distinguish between discrete events, altering how responses are aligned across time. The effect on coordination is a shift from synchronized responses to staggered or inconsistent responses, while the effect on interpretation is a reduction in temporal clarity. The system adapts to this altered structure, but the resulting behavior reflects the disruption of timing rather than the preservation of it.

Baseline and exposure shift as a result of persistent external modulation. Repeated or sustained inputs prevent full resolution of signals, leading to an upward drift in baseline signaling. Under normal conditions, signals resolve sufficiently to preserve distinct intervals between events, maintaining segmented exposure. Under distortion, exposure becomes continuous, with signals overlapping and contributing to a sustained environment of activation.

This shift reduces signal contrast and alters interpretive thresholds. When baseline is elevated, incremental changes in signaling carry less relative significance, reducing the clarity with which new signals are interpreted. The system adjusts its thresholds for response, but this adjustment changes how information is processed. The effect is a transition from discrete interpretation to continuous interpretation, with implications for coordination, partitioning, and feedback regulation.

Sensitivity adapts under these conditions as tissues adjust their responsiveness to altered signaling environments. Under normal conditions, responsiveness reflects alignment between signal and response, allowing efficient translation of information into coordinated action. Under stress-modified conditions, responsiveness shifts to accommodate changes in signal structure, altering how strongly and how quickly tissues respond.

This adaptation introduces uneven responses across tissues. Some tissues may maintain responsiveness, while others exhibit reduced or altered response patterns. The effect on coordination is increased instability, as responses no longer align consistently across the system. The effect on interpretation is a change in how signals are weighted and translated, reflecting the system's attempt to maintain function under modified conditions.

Coordination distortion emerges as these differences in responsiveness and interpretation accumulate. Under normal conditions, tissues align their responses within a shared signaling framework, producing coherent system behavior. Under distortion, divergence in interpretation leads to misalignment, with tissues responding at different times or with different intensities. This reduces overall system coherence and increases the complexity of maintaining stable outcomes.

The consequences of this distortion extend into energy routing. When coordination is disrupted, the allocation of energy across tissues reflects the divergence in responses, producing patterns that may not align with system demand. The system continues to allocate resources, but the distribution reflects altered coordination rather than optimal alignment, introducing inefficiencies into energy use and storage.

Partitioning is directly affected by these changes in coordination. Under normal conditions, allocation across use, circulation, and storage reflects coherent interpretation of signaling inputs. Under stress-modified conditions, altered interpretation leads to shifts in allocation patterns. These shifts may not correspond to immediate demand or availability, reflecting the indirect influence of external signals on energy routing.

The mismatch between allocation and demand introduces additional strain into the system. Tissues may receive or retain energy in ways that do not align with current requirements, requiring further adjustments to maintain stability. This propagation from signaling interference to partitioning illustrates how external modulation affects downstream outcomes without acting directly on allocation pathways.

Feedback loop distortion occurs as changes in timing, sensitivity, and coordination alter the relationship between signal and response. Under normal conditions, feedback loops operate with predictable timing and magnitude, allowing efficient regulation of glucose and energy availability. Under distortion, delays and mismatches in response alter the structure of these loops.

These changes produce loop instability, where corrections are delayed or exaggerated, extending the duration of adjustment cycles. The system continues to regulate, but the efficiency of regulation is reduced, and the time required to restore alignment increases. This effect demonstrates how external modulation propagates through feedback processes, altering system dynamics without directly controlling outcomes.

Variability is amplified as irregular signaling patterns emerge from these interactions. Under normal conditions, variability is constrained within structured oscillation, preserving predictability. Under distortion, irregular timing, altered baseline, and inconsistent responsiveness introduce variability that lacks structure. This reduces the predictability of system behavior and complicates interpretation across tissues.

The loss of structured oscillation affects how signals are processed. Without consistent patterns, the system cannot rely on established interpretive frameworks, increasing the range of possible responses to similar conditions. This amplification of variability reflects the cumulative effect of disrupted timing, coordination, and feedback.

Compensation interacts with these conditions by increasing signaling output in response to altered responsiveness. Under normal conditions, compensation maintains alignment between signal and response without significantly altering exposure patterns. Under stress-modified conditions, increased output contributes to elevated baseline and continuous exposure, reinforcing the conditions that necessitated compensation.

This interaction creates a feedback escalation, where increased signaling sustains elevated baseline and exposure, further altering sensitivity and coordination. The system maintains function through this adjustment, but the underlying structure of signaling becomes more complex, reflecting the layered effects of compensation and external modulation.

Hidden instability develops as the system continues to function under these altered conditions. Observable outputs may remain within functional ranges, suggesting stability, while internal dynamics shift toward increased variability, reduced clarity, and greater reliance on compensatory mechanisms. This creates a condition in which stability is maintained through altered processes that introduce structural strain.

The strain manifests as reduced resilience, with the system operating closer to the limits of its capacity to maintain alignment. Small perturbations may produce larger effects, as the system's ability to absorb variability is diminished. This hidden instability reflects the cumulative impact of external modulation on internal signaling architecture.

Failure patterns emerge when the system can no longer maintain alignment through these compensatory adjustments. Chronic misalignment of timing, sustained elevation of baseline, and persistent variability reduce the effectiveness of coordination. Feedback loops become less capable of restoring balance, and compensation reaches limits where increased output no longer produces alignment.

At this stage, the breakdown of coordination becomes more apparent, with observable instability in regulation and energy distribution. The system transitions from operating under hidden instability to exhibiting overt dysfunction, reflecting the cumulative effects of prolonged external modulation.

The Stress Interaction Mechanism integrates across all prior mechanisms, embedding external signals into the system's internal dynamics. It modifies timing, alters baseline and exposure, reshapes sensitivity and resistance, influences compensation, and amplifies variability. These effects are not isolated but interconnected, producing system-wide modulation that reflects the interaction between external inputs and internal processes.

This integration demonstrates that stress does not operate as a separate layer acting on the system from outside. It becomes part of the signaling environment, influencing how all mechanisms function. The resulting behavior reflects the full system operating under modified conditions, where external inputs are continuously integrated into internal signaling dynamics.

External signals do not override internal systems. They reshape the conditions under which those systems operate.

External signals alter internal control by reshaping how insulin signaling is interpreted, coordinated, and sustained within the system.

The Integration Mechanism

The Integration Mechanism defines how insulin signaling operates within a fully interconnected system where no single process functions independently and no outcome emerges from a single variable. Insulin does not act as an isolated regulator, nor does it operate as a central controller that directs all metabolic behavior. It exists as a coordination signal embedded within a network of interacting mechanisms, where its meaning and effect are shaped continuously by timing, sensitivity, exposure, baseline conditions, and external inputs. Integration describes the condition in which all of these variables operate simultaneously, forming a dynamic system that maintains coherence through interaction rather than through isolated control.

This integrated structure requires that signaling be understood as a continuous process rather than as a sequence of independent events. Timing determines when signals occur and how they are sequenced, sensitivity determines how they are translated into response, and baseline defines the reference state against which they are interpreted. These variables do not act separately. They intersect at every moment, shaping how insulin signaling is generated, processed, and coordinated across tissues. The resulting system behavior reflects this intersection, demonstrating that integration is not an additional layer but the condition under which all mechanisms operate.

The progression from isolated mechanisms to a unified system requires a shift in how each component is understood. Interpretation, coordination, timing, regulation, partitioning, clearance, sensitivity, resistance, compensation, exposure, baseline, variability, and input interactions were described as distinct mechanisms to establish clarity. Within the integrated system, none of these mechanisms operates independently. Each modifies the others continuously, forming a network of reciprocal influence that defines system behavior across time.

When timing interacts with exposure and baseline, the structure of signaling patterns changes, altering how signals are separated or overlap. When sensitivity interacts with compensation and resistance, the translation of signals into action is modified, influencing how tissues respond under different conditions. When variability interacts with coordination and feedback regulation, the predictability of responses shifts, affecting how the system maintains alignment. These interactions do not occur sequentially. They occur simultaneously, producing a system in which behavior emerges from the combined influence of multiple variables rather than from any single mechanism.

Insulin functions within this system as a central coordination signal, not by directing outcomes but by providing a shared informational reference point across tissues. It communicates the availability of energy and participates in aligning responses across muscle, liver, and adipose tissue. Its role is not to impose behavior but to facilitate alignment within a network of interacting variables. The meaning of insulin signaling is therefore determined by how it is interpreted within the context of timing, sensitivity, baseline, and exposure rather than by its magnitude alone.

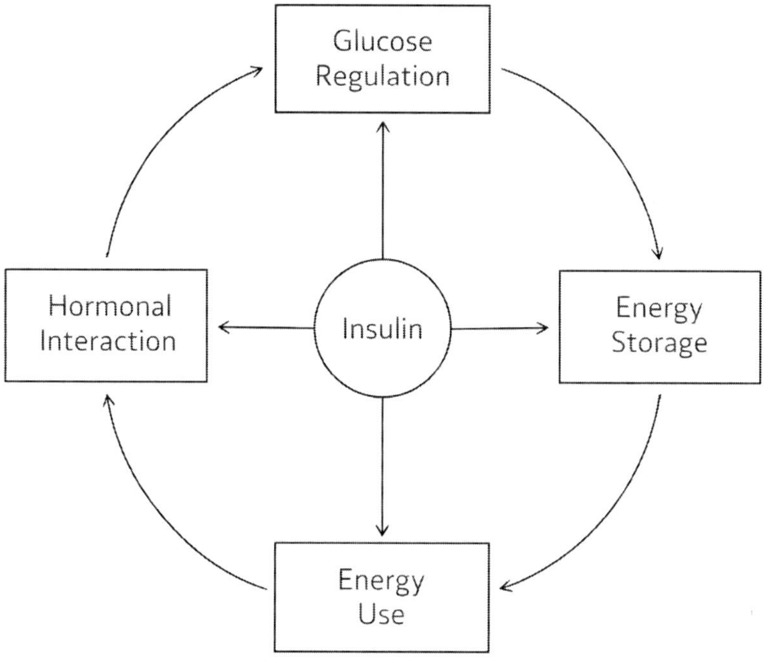

[Figure 8: Insulin as Central Coordination Signal]

This central role emerges from the way insulin integrates information across the system. Timing determines when insulin signals are initiated, sensitivity determines how those signals are translated into response, and exposure defines how they accumulate over time. Baseline conditions shape the interpretive environment, while inputs such as nutrition, fasting, and stress modify the structure of signaling patterns. Coordination arises when these variables align, allowing insulin to function as a consistent reference point across tissues. When alignment is disrupted, insulin signaling remains present, but its ability to coordinate responses is altered by the surrounding conditions.

Multi-variable coordination defines how system behavior is structured across interacting variables. Timing, sensitivity, exposure, and baseline do not operate as independent dimensions. They interact continuously, shaping how signals are generated and interpreted. For example, a signal that occurs within a low baseline environment with high sensitivity and structured timing may produce a different pattern of coordination than the same signal occurring within an elevated baseline, reduced sensitivity, and irregular timing structure. The difference does not reflect the signal itself. It reflects the interaction between variables that define the interpretive environment.

This interaction extends into how signals are distributed across tissues. Muscle, liver, and adipose tissue interpret signals based on their local conditions and their position within the system. When variables align, coordination across these tissues reflects coherent interpretation. When variables diverge, responses become misaligned, introducing variability into coordination. The system continues to function, but its behavior reflects the interaction between variables rather than the influence of any single factor.

Input interactions further demonstrate how the system operates as an integrated network. Nutrition, fasting, and stress do not act as direct drivers of metabolic outcomes. They modify the signaling environment by influencing timing, exposure, baseline, and sensitivity. These inputs alter the structure of signaling patterns, which are then interpreted within the system's current state. The effect of any input is therefore conditional, reflecting how it interacts with existing variables rather than its isolated characteristics.

Nutrition influences the magnitude and timing of signals, fasting influences the presence of low-signal intervals and baseline resolution, and stress influences the interpretive environment through external modulation. These inputs do not determine outcomes independently. They are embedded within the signaling system, contributing to patterns that shape interpretation and coordination. The resulting behavior reflects the integration of these inputs with internal mechanisms, demonstrating that outcomes emerge from interaction rather than from isolated input effects.

Temporal integration defines how signals are interpreted across time rather than within single moments. Timing, sequence, duration, and overlap determine how signals accumulate and how they are processed within the system. Past signals influence current interpretation through their effect on baseline, exposure, and sensitivity. This creates a condition in which the system operates within a continuous temporal framework, where each signal is understood in relation to prior and subsequent signals.

This temporal structure shapes how patterns are formed and how they influence system behavior. Repeated patterns of exposure alter baseline and sensitivity, which in turn affect how new signals are interpreted. Timing interacts with these variables to determine whether signals are experienced as discrete events or as components of a continuous pattern. The system therefore operates within a temporal context where patterns, rather than isolated events, define interpretation and response.

Interdependence across mechanisms defines the structure of the integrated system. Each mechanism modifies others continuously, creating a network of feedback and interaction. Timing influences exposure and baseline, which influence sensitivity and resistance, which influence compensation and coordination. Variability emerges from changes in these relationships, while inputs modify the structure of interactions. This network does not operate linearly. It reflects a system in which changes propagate across multiple layers simultaneously.

The propagation of changes illustrates how outcomes shift within the system. When baseline elevates, signal contrast decreases, affecting interpretation and coordination. When sensitivity declines, compensation increases, altering exposure and feedback regulation. When timing becomes irregular, variability increases, affecting predictability and alignment. Each change influences multiple mechanisms, demonstrating that system behavior reflects the combined effect of interacting variables rather than isolated processes.

State formation emerges from the interaction between baseline, exposure, and variability. The system does not operate within discrete events but within states defined by these variables. Baseline establishes the reference level of signaling, exposure defines how signals accumulate, and variability defines the structure of fluctuation within the system. Together, these variables create conditions under which signals are interpreted and responses are generated.

These states determine how the system behaves under different conditions. A system with low baseline, structured exposure, and low variability operates within a state that supports clear interpretation and coordination. A system with elevated baseline, continuous exposure, and high variability operates within a state that reduces clarity and increases the complexity of coordination. The system's behavior reflects the state in which it operates, demonstrating that outcomes are shaped by the interaction of multiple variables rather than by individual signals.

Stability emerges as a property of alignment across these variables. It is not controlled directly and does not result from optimizing any single component. Stability reflects the coherence of interactions between timing, sensitivity, exposure, baseline, and coordination. When these variables align, the system maintains consistent interpretation and coordinated response. When they diverge, instability emerges as a result of misalignment rather than as a failure of any single mechanism.

This emergent property requires continuous maintenance rather than discrete achievement. The system adjusts constantly to changing conditions, integrating new signals and modifying responses to preserve alignment. Stability is therefore dynamic, reflecting the system's capacity to maintain coherence under variability rather than to eliminate variability entirely.

Instability emerges from multi-variable breakdown rather than from single-point failure. Misalignment between timing, sensitivity, exposure, and baseline introduces distortion into interpretation and coordination. These distortions compound as they propagate across mechanisms, affecting feedback regulation, partitioning, and variability. The system may continue to function, but its behavior reflects the cumulative effect of misalignment rather than the influence of any single factor.

This multi-variable breakdown demonstrates the limitation of reductionist models. Approaches that focus on individual variables such as spikes, inputs, or sensitivity fail to capture the complexity of the system. A single variable cannot define system behavior because outcomes emerge from the interaction between multiple variables operating simultaneously. Spike-focused models overlook exposure and baseline, input-focused models overlook interpretation and coordination, and sensitivity-focused models overlook timing and variability.

Predictability is therefore limited by the number of interacting variables within the system. As variables increase, the range of possible outcomes expands, and behavior becomes conditional rather than deterministic. The system operates within ranges defined by interaction rather than producing fixed outcomes from specific inputs. This does not imply randomness. It reflects the complexity of a system in which multiple variables interact continuously across time.

Adaptive system behavior emerges from this complexity. The system does not maintain a fixed equilibrium but operates within a moving window of stability defined by changing conditions. Timing, sensitivity, exposure, and baseline shift in response to inputs and internal dynamics, and the system adjusts accordingly. This adaptation preserves function within a range of conditions, demonstrating that stability is maintained through flexibility rather than through fixed control.

System boundaries define the limits within which this adaptation can occur. Capacity constraints, threshold effects, and non-linear transitions shape how the system responds to changes in variables. When interactions remain within these boundaries, the system maintains stability through adjustment. When they exceed these limits, transitions occur that alter system behavior more substantially. These transitions reflect the non-linear nature of the system, where small changes in variables can produce larger shifts when thresholds are crossed.

Full-system synthesis integrates all mechanisms into a unified model in which insulin signaling is embedded within a network of interacting variables. Timing, sensitivity, exposure, baseline, variability, and inputs operate simultaneously, shaping how signals are interpreted and how responses are coordinated. The behavior of the system reflects this integration, demonstrating that outcomes emerge from the interaction of mechanisms rather than from isolated processes.

This synthesis establishes that insulin is not an isolated regulator but a component of a broader signaling architecture. Its role is defined by how it interacts with other variables, providing a reference point for coordination while being influenced by the conditions under which it operates. The system functions as a whole, with each mechanism contributing to the overall pattern of behavior.

Stability is not controlled by one variable. It emerges from the alignment of many.

Metabolic stability is not the result of controlling individual signals, but of maintaining alignment across a system of interacting variables that operate continuously across time.

The Stability Threshold Mechanism

The Stability Threshold Mechanism defines how metabolic stability operates within bounded ranges rather than fixed states, and how these ranges establish the limits within which coordinated signaling remains functional. Stability is not a binary condition in which the system is either stable or unstable. It exists within tolerance ranges defined by the interaction of timing, sensitivity, baseline, exposure, and variability. A threshold represents the boundary at which these interacting variables can no longer maintain alignment, and where system behavior transitions from structured coordination to increasing distortion.

Within this framework, a threshold is not a single point but a boundary region shaped by multiple variables operating together. Timing determines the structure of signaling sequences, baseline defines the reference level for interpretation, and sensitivity governs how signals are translated into response. When these variables operate within compatible ranges, the system maintains coherence. As they approach their limits, the interaction between them begins to compress, reducing flexibility and narrowing the range within which coordinated behavior can be sustained.

Stability is therefore expressed as a range rather than a point. There is no fixed optimal state to which the system returns. Instead, the system operates within a window of acceptable variation defined by the interaction of multiple variables. Baseline may fluctuate within a range that preserves signal contrast, timing may vary within a structure that maintains sequence integrity, and sensitivity may adjust within limits that allow consistent signal translation. These variations do not disrupt stability as long as they remain within the system's tolerance ranges.

As variation approaches the boundaries of these ranges, the nature of system behavior begins to change. The same degree of fluctuation that is accommodated within the central range becomes more consequential near the edges. Timing irregularities may begin to overlap, baseline elevation may reduce signal distinction, and sensitivity shifts may alter response consistency. The system remains functional, but its capacity to absorb variation decreases, reflecting the approach toward a threshold.

Multi-variable tolerance defines how these ranges combine to produce overall system capacity. Each variable—timing, baseline, sensitivity, exposure, and variability—has its own tolerance range. These ranges do not operate independently. They overlap and interact, creating a composite tolerance that defines the system's ability to maintain alignment. A narrowing in one variable's range can be offset by stability in another, allowing the system to remain within its overall tolerance.

This interaction introduces the possibility of compensation across variables. When timing becomes less structured, increased sensitivity or reduced baseline may preserve coordination. When baseline elevates, more precise timing or reduced variability may maintain interpretive clarity. These trade-offs allow the system to operate within its tolerance range even as individual variables approach their boundaries. However, as more variables compress simultaneously, the capacity for compensation diminishes, and the system approaches a threshold.

Approaching a threshold is characterized by gradual misalignment rather than abrupt change. Timing may become slightly irregular, baseline may drift upward, and variability may increase within a range that still supports function. These changes do not immediately produce instability. They reflect the system operating closer to its limits, where flexibility is reduced and adjustments require greater coordination across variables.

As tolerance compresses, the system's ability to absorb variation decreases. Small deviations in timing, baseline, or sensitivity produce more pronounced effects on coordination and interpretation. The system continues to function, but the margin within which it can maintain alignment becomes narrower. This reduction in flexibility reflects the system's proximity to a threshold, where the interaction between variables becomes more constrained.

Early indicators of this proximity appear as changes in variability, signal clarity, and coordination timing. Variability may increase as signaling patterns become less structured, baseline elevation may reduce contrast between signals, and coordination may exhibit slight delays or inconsistencies. These indicators reflect the system's attempt to maintain alignment within a compressed range, where adjustments are more frequent and less efficient.

Signal degradation emerges near the threshold as interpretive precision declines. When baseline is elevated and variability is increased, the distinction between signals becomes less clear. Sensitivity adjustments may alter signal translation, and feedback loops may become less efficient in maintaining alignment. These changes do not eliminate signaling function but reduce the clarity with which signals are interpreted and coordinated.

At the boundary, compensation becomes more prominent as the system attempts to maintain function under constrained conditions. Increased signaling output may offset reduced sensitivity, extended exposure may compensate for irregular timing, and altered coordination may preserve overall function despite local misalignment. These compensatory adjustments reflect the system operating at the limits of its tolerance, where maintaining alignment requires greater effort across variables.

This compensatory state narrows the system's margin further. As compensation increases, baseline may elevate, exposure may become more continuous, and variability may increase. These changes reinforce the conditions that required compensation, creating a feedback interaction that reduces flexibility. The system remains within its tolerance range, but the range itself becomes more constrained, reflecting proximity to the threshold.

The hidden instability zone emerges within this compressed range, where the system continues to function but operates under increased structural strain. Coordination is maintained, but alignment requires continuous adjustment across timing, sensitivity, and baseline. Variability increases, but remains within limits that preserve overall function. The system appears stable, yet its capacity to absorb additional variation is reduced.

Within this zone, resilience is diminished. Small changes in input, timing, or responsiveness produce larger effects than they would within a wider tolerance range. The system's ability to maintain structured oscillation is compromised, and its reliance on compensatory mechanisms increases. This reflects a condition in which stability is maintained through constrained interaction rather than through flexible alignment.

Threshold crossing represents a transition in which the system moves beyond its tolerance range. At this boundary, the system does not respond proportionally to additional change. The same incremental shift that was previously absorbed within tolerance now produces a disproportionate effect on coordination and interpretation. This transition is non-linear, reflecting the interaction of multiple variables reaching their limits simultaneously. A small change in timing, baseline, or sensitivity can produce a larger shift in system behavior when the system is at its boundary. Coordination may be disrupted, feedback loops may become unstable, and variability may increase beyond structured limits.

This transition is not defined by a single variable exceeding its range. It reflects the combined effect of multiple variables interacting beyond their collective tolerance. Timing irregularities may overlap with elevated baseline and reduced sensitivity, producing a condition in which signals can no longer be interpreted consistently. The system transitions from constrained stability to a state where alignment cannot be maintained.

Post-threshold behavior reflects persistent misalignment across variables. Feedback loops may operate with delayed or exaggerated responses, coordination across tissues may become inconsistent, and variability may increase beyond structured oscillation. The system continues to function, but its behavior reflects a different state, where signals are interpreted within a distorted environment.

These changes illustrate that thresholds are dynamic rather than fixed. The tolerance ranges that define stability shift over time, influenced by exposure patterns, baseline conditions, sensitivity adjustments, and input interactions. A system that operates within a certain range under one set of conditions may operate within a different range under another, reflecting the adaptive nature of the system.

This dynamic nature extends to system capacity limits. The system's ability to compensate, adjust, and maintain alignment is finite, defined by structural constraints within timing, sensitivity, baseline, and coordination. These limits do not represent fixed boundaries but ranges that can expand or contract depending on system conditions. As these limits are approached, the system's flexibility decreases, reflecting the narrowing of tolerance. This capacity is finite, and as it is approached, the system's ability to maintain alignment through adjustment diminishes.

Interdependence becomes more pronounced at these boundaries. A shift in one variable influences others more strongly, producing cascading effects across the system. Elevated baseline affects sensitivity and timing, altered timing affects variability and coordination, and changes in sensitivity affect compensation and exposure. These interactions amplify the effects of individual changes, demonstrating that no variable operates in isolation at the threshold.

Predictability decreases as the system approaches and crosses its threshold. Within stable ranges, the system produces responses that are consistent within a defined pattern. Near the boundary, increased variability and reduced clarity expand the range of possible outcomes. The system becomes more sensitive to perturbation, reflecting the interaction of compressed tolerance ranges across variables.

This sensitivity does not imply randomness but reflects the complexity of multi-variable interaction under constrained conditions. Timing, baseline, and sensitivity interact in ways that produce a wider range of responses to similar inputs. The system continues to operate within a defined structure, but that structure becomes less predictable as tolerance narrows.

The Stability Threshold Mechanism integrates directly with the full system model by applying constraints to all prior mechanisms. Timing, sensitivity, exposure, baseline, variability, and input interactions all operate within tolerance ranges that define stability. These ranges interact continuously, shaping how signals are interpreted and how responses are coordinated across tissues.

This integration demonstrates that stability is not defined by the absence of variability or the presence of optimal conditions. It is defined by the system's ability to operate within ranges that preserve structured interaction between variables. As long as these interactions remain within tolerance, the system maintains coherence. When they approach or exceed their boundaries, the nature of system behavior changes, reflecting the transition from structured variability to increasing instability.

Systems do not operate indefinitely.

They operate within limits.

Metabolic systems do not maintain stability by eliminating variability, but by operating within the limits that allow variability to remain structured, interpretable, and coordinated across time.

The Long-Term Drift Mechanism

The Long-Term Drift Mechanism defines how metabolic systems gradually reposition over time through the accumulation of small, individually tolerable deviations across interacting variables. This process does not represent a discrete failure or a sudden loss of stability. It reflects a progressive shift in system structure, where alignment across timing, baseline, exposure, sensitivity, variability, and coordination is incrementally altered. The system continues to function throughout this process, maintaining output while the internal conditions that support that output are slowly reconfigured.

Drift is not an immediate expression of instability. It is a condition in which minor misalignments persist and compound, altering how signals are interpreted and coordinated without producing immediate disruption. The system does not recognize drift as failure in real time because each individual deviation remains within tolerance. However, as these deviations accumulate, the structure of signaling changes, reducing the system's capacity to maintain stable coordination under variability. Compensation increases, baseline may shift, and variability may expand, all while function appears preserved.

Stability degrades incrementally under drift. There is no single moment at which the system transitions from stable to unstable. Early drift is effectively invisible within the system's tolerance ranges. Timing irregularities remain within acceptable limits, baseline fluctuations preserve sufficient contrast, and sensitivity adjustments maintain response alignment. The system operates within its range, and the structural changes occurring beneath this operation do not produce immediate observable disruption.

As drift progresses, the system requires increasing adjustment to maintain alignment. Mid-phase drift is characterized by a greater reliance on compensation, where signaling output adjusts to preserve coordination despite underlying shifts in responsiveness and timing. Variability may increase, and feedback loops may require more extended cycles to maintain regulation. The system remains functional, but the effort required to maintain that function increases, reflecting a reduction in structural efficiency.

In later stages, drift produces constrained stability. The system continues to operate within its tolerance range, but that range has narrowed. Timing may exhibit more frequent misalignment, baseline may remain elevated, and variability may approach the limits of structured oscillation. The system appears stable while becoming less capable of remaining stable, as the margin for absorbing additional variation diminishes.

This progression is driven by the accumulation of small deviations rather than by large, isolated changes. Each deviation—whether a slight alteration in timing, a minor elevation in baseline, a small increase in variability, or a subtle shift in sensitivity—remains within tolerance when considered independently. No single deviation produces instability. However, the accumulation of these deviations alters the system's position within its tolerance ranges, moving it gradually toward the boundary.

The effect of accumulation is not additive in a simple sense. It is structural. As deviations accumulate, they interact with one another, altering how variables influence each other. Slight timing irregularities may increase overlap between signals, contributing to baseline elevation. Baseline elevation may reduce signal contrast, altering sensitivity. Changes in sensitivity may require increased signaling output, affecting exposure. These interactions propagate across the system, demonstrating that stability is not lost from magnitude but from accumulation.

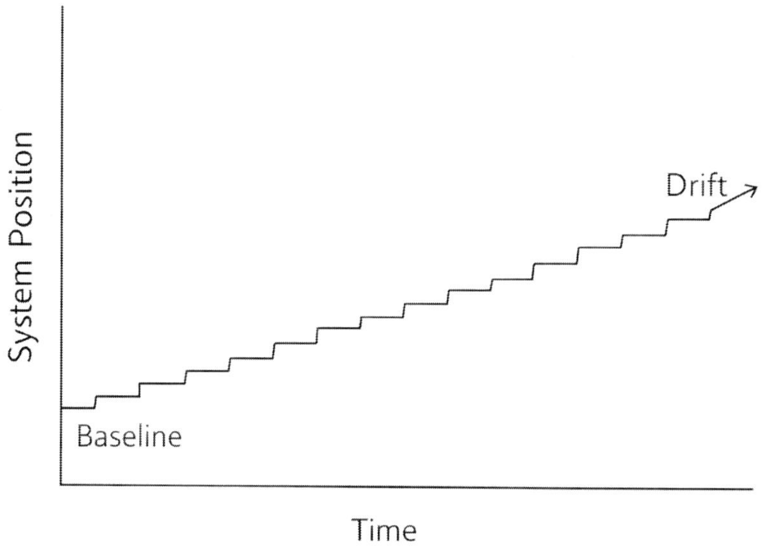

[Figure 9: Gradual Drift Over Time]

Drift must be distinguished from random variability. Variability represents fluctuation within a structured range, where oscillations maintain coherence and interpretive clarity. Drift represents directional change in the system's position within that range. It is not oscillation around a stable point but a gradual repositioning of that point itself. Baseline may shift upward over time, timing may become progressively less structured, and sensitivity may adjust in a consistent direction, altering how signals are translated.

This directional movement changes the interpretive environment. Signals that once occurred within a low baseline environment with clear temporal separation may now occur within an elevated baseline with reduced contrast. The meaning of those signals changes as a result of this shift, even if their magnitude remains similar. The system's trajectory therefore determines how signals are interpreted, demonstrating that drift reshapes meaning across time.

A critical distinction within this process is between temporary variation and structural change. Temporary variation resolves within the system's existing structure. Timing irregularities may occur but are followed by periods of alignment. Baseline may fluctuate but returns to prior levels. Sensitivity may adjust but reverts within its established range. These variations do not accumulate and therefore do not alter the system's position.

Structural drift persists and compounds. Deviations do not fully resolve, and their effects carry forward into subsequent signaling conditions. Baseline may remain slightly elevated, timing may retain minor misalignment, and sensitivity may continue to shift. These changes are incorporated into the system's ongoing operation, altering future interpretation. The system does not just experience change; it stores change, embedding prior deviations into its current state.

Drift propagates across variables rather than remaining localized. Timing drift alters the sequence and spacing of signals, increasing the likelihood of overlap. This overlap contributes to baseline drift, as signals do not fully resolve. Baseline drift alters exposure, increasing cumulative signaling load. Increased exposure influences sensitivity, gradually shifting responsiveness. Sensitivity drift affects coordination, as tissues interpret signals differently. Variability drift emerges as oscillation becomes less structured, reflecting the combined effect of these changes.

This propagation demonstrates that drift is not confined to a single mechanism. It is a system-wide process that emerges from the interaction of multiple variables over time. Each variable contributes to the trajectory, and changes in one variable influence others, creating a network of interdependent shifts that reposition the system gradually.

Compensation plays a central role in allowing drift to continue without detection. As sensitivity shifts and coordination becomes less precise, the system increases signaling output to maintain functional alignment. This increased output preserves observable stability, ensuring that responses remain within functional ranges despite underlying structural change. Compensation therefore masks the progression of drift by maintaining output while allowing internal conditions to shift.

This masking effect reinforces drift. Increased signaling output contributes to baseline elevation and sustained exposure, which further influences sensitivity and timing. The system adapts to these conditions, incorporating them into its operation. Compensation does not halt drift. It allows drift to proceed while maintaining the appearance of stability, extending the period during which structural changes accumulate.

Hidden instability emerges within this phase of drift. The system continues to produce coordinated outputs, and feedback regulation remains functional within observable ranges. However, the internal structure supporting these outputs has shifted. Timing may be less precise, baseline may be elevated, variability may be increased, and coordination may require continuous adjustment. The system appears stable, but the conditions that define stability have changed.

This hidden instability reflects a divergence between appearance and structure. The system maintains function through compensation and adaptation, but the underlying alignment between variables is reduced. The capacity to absorb additional variation is diminished, and the system operates closer to its threshold. This condition is not recognized as failure because outputs remain within expected ranges, yet it represents a progression toward reduced stability.

Drift establishes the pathway toward threshold crossing. Thresholds represent the boundaries of tolerance ranges, where the system can no longer maintain alignment across variables. Drift moves the system toward these boundaries by gradually compressing tolerance. Timing irregularities accumulate, baseline elevates, sensitivity shifts, and variability increases, all contributing to a reduction in flexibility.

The system does not cross a threshold randomly. It is positioned there through accumulated drift across time. When the system reaches the boundary, a relatively small additional deviation can produce a larger shift in behavior due to the compressed tolerance range. The transition appears sudden, but it reflects the cumulative effect of prior drift rather than an isolated event.

Feedback loops are altered as drift progresses. Under stable conditions, feedback operates with consistent timing and magnitude, allowing efficient correction of deviations. As drift alters timing, baseline, and sensitivity, feedback becomes less precise. Corrections may be delayed, responses may be exaggerated, and adjustment cycles may extend over longer durations. These changes reflect the system's adaptation to a shifting interpretive environment.

The inefficiency of feedback reinforces drift. Delayed corrections allow deviations to persist longer, contributing to accumulation. Exaggerated responses may overshoot, introducing additional variability. Extended cycles increase exposure duration, affecting baseline and sensitivity. Feedback loops continue to function, but their altered structure contributes to the progression of drift rather than fully counteracting it.

Reversibility changes as drift advances. In early stages, deviations are more easily resolved because the system remains within a wider tolerance range. Timing can realign, baseline can return toward prior levels, and sensitivity can adjust within its range. As drift becomes more advanced, these deviations become embedded within the system's structure. The system adapts to the new conditions, incorporating them into its baseline operation.

This adaptation reduces the system's reference to its prior state. The elevated baseline becomes the new baseline, altered timing becomes the new timing structure, and shifted sensitivity becomes the new responsiveness range. The system forgets its prior state in the sense that it no longer operates relative to it. This does not imply permanence, but it reflects a change in the system's operating position, where prior conditions no longer define interpretation.

Failure patterns emerge as the endpoint of drift rather than as a separate process. Prolonged compensation maintains output under increasingly constrained conditions, elevated baseline persists, variability increases beyond structured oscillation, and coordination declines. These patterns reflect the cumulative effect of drift across variables, demonstrating that failure is not an abrupt event but the continuation of a long-term process.

This framing leads to a critical distinction between system position and system events. Outcomes are not determined by isolated events but reflect the position of the system within its tolerance ranges. A given input or signal may produce different outcomes depending on whether the system is operating within a stable range or near its threshold. Drift determines this position by gradually repositioning the system over time.

The implication is that system behavior cannot be understood by examining individual events in isolation. It must be understood in relation to the accumulated changes that define the system's current state. Drift provides the mechanism by which these changes occur, linking time, accumulation, and eventual instability into a continuous process.

Drift precedes failure. What appears as sudden instability reflects the culmination of gradual change that has repositioned the system beyond its capacity to maintain alignment. The system does not fail in the moment it becomes unstable. It fails after a prolonged process of drift that repositions it beyond its capacity to maintain coordination across interacting variables.

The Insulin Stability Synthesis

The Insulin Stability Synthesis is the integrated model through which metabolic stability emerges from the interaction of core signaling dimensions across time. This model does not position insulin as a controller, a driver, or a target. It positions insulin as a coordination signal within a system whose behavior is shaped by the relationships among multiple variables operating simultaneously. Stability is not produced by any single variable, any single signal, or any isolated mechanism. It is produced through alignment across interacting variables that continuously influence one another within the constraints of time, state, and system capacity.

This synthesis requires a shift from isolated explanation to unified operation. Earlier mechanisms clarified distinct aspects of system behavior by separating interpretation from timing, coordination from partitioning, clearance from exposure, and sensitivity from resistance. That separation was useful for analytical precision, but it does not reflect how the system operates in real conditions. In real operation, there is no timing mechanism functioning independently of baseline, no sensitivity mechanism functioning independently of exposure, and no coordination mechanism functioning independently of interpretation. There is only system behavior. It emerges from the simultaneous interaction among variables that are always active together.

The transition from mechanisms to system therefore changes the level of explanation. Instead of asking what each mechanism does on its own, the relevant question becomes how these variables interact in the same moment to shape signaling meaning and response. Timing interacts with clearance to determine whether signals remain distinct or overlap. Overlap influences exposure, exposure influences baseline, and baseline influences signal clarity. Signal clarity shapes how tissues interpret insulin, and tissue interpretation determines whether coordination remains coherent. The system does not move linearly from one mechanism to the next. It operates as a network in which each variable modifies the conditions under which the others function.

Within this integrated model, several core signaling dimensions define the structure of operation. Signal clarity refers to the system's ability to distinguish one signaling state from another. It depends on the relationship between baseline and variability, because elevated baseline and disorganized fluctuation reduce contrast between signals. Timing refers to sequence, spacing, and overlap, shaping whether signals are experienced as discrete events or as parts of continuous exposure. Sensitivity defines how effectively signals are translated into response, while clearance defines how long signals persist and whether they resolve sufficiently to preserve separation.

Exposure describes the cumulative signaling load the system experiences across time, and baseline defines the reference state against which new signals are interpreted. Coordination refers to the alignment of responses across tissues, where muscle, liver, and adipose tissue participate within a shared signaling environment. These dimensions are not separate components assembled after the fact. They are dimensions of the same system. A change in one dimension alters the interpretive conditions of the others. Reduced clearance changes exposure, altered exposure shifts baseline, elevated baseline reduces clarity, reduced clarity influences sensitivity and coordination, and the resulting responses feed back into future signaling patterns.

This structure leads to a pattern-based model of metabolic regulation. The system does not operate on isolated events, discrete spikes, or singular moments of signaling. It operates on patterns across time. A signaling pattern is composed of magnitude, duration, frequency, sequence, and overlap. No single one of these defines the pattern alone. A signal of moderate magnitude but prolonged duration contributes differently to system behavior than a brief signal of higher magnitude. Frequent signals with incomplete resolution create a different environment than less frequent signals with clear separation. The system interprets patterns, not events. Events are observable. Patterns are operative.

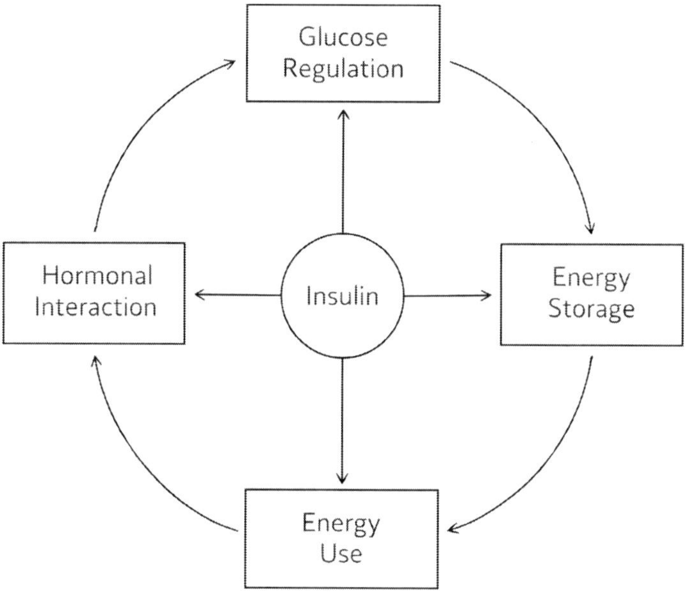

[Figure 8: Insulin as Central Coordination Signal]

Because the system interprets patterns, it cannot be understood through event-based reasoning alone. A spike in isolation does not define system state, just as a single deviation does not define drift. Meaning arises from the arrangement of signals across time and from the conditions under which they are interpreted. This is why baseline, exposure, and timing matter as much as magnitude. The system is not responding to individual moments in a vacuum. It is responding to the structured relationships between signals, within a history of prior signals and within a current state shaped by cumulative exposure and variable alignment.

Interpretation sits at the center of this model because signals function as information rather than as direct causes. Insulin does not force outcomes into existence. It provides information about energy availability within a broader signaling environment, and tissues respond by interpreting that information relative to their roles, current demands, and prior conditions. Muscle interprets insulin through utilization and uptake, the liver through circulation and regulation, and adipose tissue through buffering and allocation. Behavior is not the signal itself. Behavior is the interpreted response to the signal within system state.

This distinction changes how outcomes are understood. Outcomes do not reflect the mere presence of insulin. They reflect how insulin signaling is interpreted under particular conditions of baseline, exposure, timing, and sensitivity. The same signal can produce different responses depending on whether it emerges from a low baseline or an elevated one, whether it occurs in a structured sequence or within irregular overlap, and whether tissues remain responsive or are operating under reduced sensitivity with compensatory signaling. Interpretation is therefore not an accessory to regulation. It is the core function through which signaling becomes system behavior.

Insulin must also be positioned neutrally within this system. It is not inherently beneficial or harmful, and it is not properly understood through moral or evaluative framing. Insulin is neutral information.

It reflects energy availability, coordinates distribution, and participates in aligning tissues within the signaling environment. Its function is informational and relational rather than directional in a simple causal sense. Distortion does not arise from insulin itself. It arises when the signaling environment in which insulin operates becomes altered, when interpretation loses clarity, and when variables that support coordinated response become misaligned.

This neutrality is essential because it prevents the system from being reduced to a single explanatory object. If insulin is treated as the cause of outcomes, the rest of the system disappears from view. But problems do not arise from insulin in isolation. They emerge from the interaction between elevated baseline, altered exposure, reduced sensitivity, distorted timing, increased variability, impaired clearance, and tissue-level misalignment. Insulin participates in these conditions, but it does not independently create them. The system creates its own behavior through the way variables interact around the signal.

Stability within this synthesis can therefore be defined precisely as alignment across variables. Stability exists when timing preserves structured sequence, when clearance allows meaningful resolution, when exposure remains interpretable, when baseline preserves contrast, when variability remains structured, when sensitivity supports efficient translation, and when tissues remain coordinated in their responses. In this state, signals remain clear enough to be distinguished, responses remain coherent enough to support regulation, and adjustment remains efficient enough to preserve system function across changing conditions.

Misalignment produces the opposite condition. Signals lose clarity when elevated baseline and variability reduce distinction. Responses diverge when timing becomes irregular and sensitivity varies across tissues. Exposure may become continuous rather than segmented, and compensation may preserve output while distorting underlying structure. In this state, instability is not a sudden event. It is a system condition in which the relationships between variables no longer support consistent interpretation and coordinated response. High baseline combined with low sensitivity, irregular timing combined with high exposure, or compensation combined with reduced signal clarity are not isolated problems. They are examples of system-wide misalignment.

Time is the primary dimension through which these relationships become meaningful. The system is path-dependent, meaning its current state reflects prior signaling conditions rather than merely present inputs. Past exposure influences baseline, baseline influences interpretation, interpretation influences response, and response shapes future signaling patterns. Drift occurs because small deviations are stored rather than erased, and threshold crossing occurs because those accumulated deviations reposition the system over time. Without time, there is no exposure, no baseline formation, no compensation, and no drift. Time is the dimension through which patterns become states.

System state can therefore be modeled as a function of baseline, exposure, and variability. Baseline provides the reference state, exposure defines cumulative signaling load, and variability defines the structure of fluctuation around that state. Together, these variables shape the environment within which signals are interpreted. State determines interpretation, and interpretation determines response. Inputs do not determine outcomes on their own. State determines how inputs are translated into outcomes because the same input modifies different systems differently depending on their existing baseline, exposure profile, and variability structure.

This is why nutrition, fasting, and stress must be understood as modifiers rather than drivers. Nutrition changes signaling patterns by affecting timing, magnitude, and duration. Fasting changes signaling patterns by altering baseline resolution, exposure segmentation, and signal separation. Stress changes signaling patterns by modifying the interpretive environment, temporal structure, and responsiveness across tissues. These inputs do not directly create outcomes. They influence the system through pattern modification. Their significance depends on the state into which they enter and the alignment of variables already operating there.

Feedback loops provide the mechanism of continuous adjustment within this model. The system is never static. It continuously compares current conditions with ongoing signaling information and adjusts response accordingly. When alignment is preserved, feedback remains efficient: timing is coherent, sensitivity is sufficient, and corrections occur without excessive delay or overshoot. When alignment is reduced, feedback becomes less precise. Corrections may be delayed, exaggerated, or prolonged because baseline, exposure, and sensitivity have altered the conditions under which feedback operates. The system continues adjusting, but the quality of adjustment depends on the structure of variable alignment.

These processes operate within limits. Stability is maintained within bounds, not indefinitely and not without constraint. Tolerance is finite because timing can only become so irregular before sequence loses meaning, baseline can only elevate so far before contrast collapses, exposure can only accumulate so much before continuous signaling changes state, and compensation can only increase so much before it reinforces the distortions it is preserving against. Stability is therefore not the elimination of all deviation. It is the capacity to maintain interpretability and coordination within system limits.

The complete system model can be reconstructed as a continuous loop. Inputs modify signaling patterns. Those patterns create exposure and shape baseline. Baseline, exposure, and variability establish system state. State shapes how signals are interpreted across tissues. Interpretation drives response through sensitivity and coordination. Response then feeds back into future signaling conditions, altering subsequent exposure, baseline, and interpretive context. This loop is continuous, and its operation across time produces both stability and instability depending on the degree of alignment among its variables.

Within this loop, insulin remains central but not dominant in a simplistic sense. It is central because it functions as a shared coordination signal through which energy availability is communicated across tissues. It is not dominant because its meaning and effect are always conditional on timing, clearance, exposure, baseline, variability, sensitivity, and inputs. The system does not revolve around insulin as a controlling force. It uses insulin as a reference signal within a broader pattern-based architecture of interpretation and response.

The final synthesis is therefore clear. Insulin is part of a system, not a self-explaining variable. Stability is emergent rather than imposed. Behavior is pattern-based rather than event-based. Outcomes are conditional rather than absolute. The system operates through interacting dimensions whose alignment determines whether signaling remains interpretable, responses remain coordinated, and regulation remains structurally stable across time.

Metabolic stability is not achieved by controlling individual signals. It is maintained through the alignment of signaling patterns across time within a system of interacting variables.

Insulin does not determine outcomes. It participates in a system that does.

About the Author

Nathan Reed writes about metabolic stability in systems exposed to load, variability, and time.

His work examines how biological capacity is shaped by energy availability, recovery architecture, sleep amplitude, muscle mass, environmental demand and workload. Rather than treating nutrition, fasting, sleep, and training as isolated tactics, he approaches them as interacting regulatory systems governed by margin, buffering, oscillatory coherence, and constraint dominance.

The Stability framework explores how physiological compression accumulates gradually and how proportional calibration preserves long-horizon resilience across decades. The objective is not peak optimization, but preservation of functional continuity under load.

Insulin Stability is part of a broader metabolic stability ecosystem developed under Perennial Publishing, each volume addressing a distinct vector of biological durability.

The work is designed for readers who prefer structural clarity over motivational rhetoric and long-horizon coherence over short-term intensity.

The Metabolic Stability Series

Metabolic Stability: *A Systems Guide to Blood Sugar, Fasting, and Long-Term Metabolic Health*

(Cornerstone Volume)

Fasting Fundamentals: *A Systems Guide to Metabolic Flexibility, Fat Loss, and Long-Term Health*

(Foundational Volume)

Intermittent Fasting: *Metabolic Timing, Body Composition, and Sustainable Health*

Prolonged Fasting: *A Systems Guide to Duration, Recovery, and Metabolic Limits*

Electrolytes: *A Systems Guide to Hydration, Electrolyte Balance, and Physiological Stability*

Insulin Stability: ***Blood Sugar, Insulin Resistance, and Metabolic Health***

Future Titles Include:
Glucose Stability
Energy Stability
Adaptation and Drift

The Vitality Series:
Sleep and Recovery
Strength and Aging
Hormones & Sexual Health

Part of a Broader Stability Framework

The Metabolic Stability Series is part of a larger stability ecosystem published by Perennial Publishing.

Related domains include:

Money Stability — structural durability in financial systems

Career Stability — positioning, load tolerance, and transition resilience

Mental Stability — cognitive steadiness under pressure and uncertainty

Emotional Stability — regulatory steadiness in environments that do not slow down

Foundations — low-fragility life architecture

Vitality — energy, strength, and biological function across time

Each domain approaches stability as a structural problem: capacity versus load, buffering versus shock, governance versus drift. Together, they form a unified framework for long-horizon durability across the major systems that shape human trajectory.

About Perennial Publishing

Perennial Publishing produces practical systems guides for building stability in an unstable world.

Our books explore the foundations of long-term resilience across health, finance, career, and everyday decision-making. Each title focuses on clear frameworks, durable principles, and practical strategies that help readers build lasting stability rather than short-term fixes.

The Perennial catalog includes series on metabolic health, financial stability, career systems, and personal consistency. While each book stands on its own, they share a common goal: helping individuals create durable systems that support a stable and sustainable life.

Made in United States
North Haven, CT
04 November 2026

21768644R00088